Multiple Choice Questions in Pathology for the FRCS

Multiple Choice Questions in Pathology for the FRCS

James McDiarmid FRCS
Jason Bernard FRCS
Tamsin Greenwell
Alan Li FRCS
Nick Marshall FRCS
Chris Thurnell
Chris Stone FRCS

Edward Arnold
A member of the Hodder Headline Group
LONDON BOSTON SYDNEY AUCKLAND

First published in Great Britain 1995 by
Edward Arnold, a division of Hodder Headline PLC,
338 Euston Road, London NW1 3BH

© 1995 Edward Arnold

Distributed in the Americas by Little, Brown and Company,
34 Beacon Street, Boston, MA 02108

All rights reserved. No part of this publication may be reproduced or transmitted in any form or by any means, electronically or mechanically, including photocopying, recording or any information storage or retrieval system, without the prior permission in writing from the publisher or a licence permitting restricted copying. In the United Kingdom such licences are issued by the Copyright Licensing Agency: 90 Tottenham Court Road, London W1P 9HE.

Whilst the advice and information in this book is believed to be true and accurate at the date of going to press, neither the authors nor the publisher can accept any legal responsibility or liability for any errors or omissions that may be made.

British Library Cataloguing in Publication Data
A catalogue record for this book is available from the British Library

Library of Congress Cataloging-in-Publication Data
A catalog record for this book is available from the Library of Congress

ISBN 0-340-59435-7

1 2 3 4 5   95 96 97 98 99

Produced by Gray Publishing, Tunbridge Wells, Kent
Printed and bound in Great Britain by J. W. Arrowsmith Ltd, Bristol

Contents

Preface	vii
1 Inflammation and the immune system	1
2 The pathology of shock	13
3 Cardiac, vascular and respiratory pathology	19
4 Gastrointestinal and hepatobiliary pathology	25
5 Renal pathology	29
6 Fracture healing and the musculoskeletal system	33
7 The endocrine system	37
8 Haematology	41
9 CNS pathology	49
10 Microbiology, sterilization and disinfection	53
11 Oncology	63

PREFACE

The authors met whilst employed as anatomy demonstrators at the University of Manchester. After several barbecues and much revision they noticed the lack of a good MCQ revision book for the part A FRCS. Having passed the exam their attentions were turned to producing such a text which three years later has been published in the form of MCQs in anatomy, physiology and pathology for the FRCS.

The part FRCS has a reputation for being the toughest of all postgraduate examinations; whether this reputation is justified is debatable, however the scope of the applied basic sciences part of the examination is unarguably vast. With a recent change in the format of the exam even more emphasis has been placed on MCQs as a way of assessing candidates' knowledge. Both the style and the depth of question encountered in the primary have been recreated by seven authors who between them have passed the primary FRCS examinations of all three UK Colleges of Surgeons. It is also true that a large amount of the syllabuses of the FRCS and the MRCOG overlap and it is hoped that these books will also be found useful in this area. Detailed explanations to each answer are provided and it is hoped that readers will find these both unambiguous and educational.

The importance of focused revision cannot be overemphasized and these books are in no way supposed to take the place of the usual learning texts (listed below) and cadaveric dissection, indeed their roles lie in the final preparation for the exam once the bulk of reading has been done. We hope that these books will not only help in polishing exam technique but also clarify some of the important factual points that they initially found confusing.

Optimal MCQ examination technique varies considerably between candidates and the number of questions left unanswered in a negative marking MCQ test depends very much upon both one's core knowledge and the degree to which one is prepared to gamble if unsure of the answer. It is recommended that candidates experiment for themselves in order to elucidate what percentage of answered questions gives them the overall best mark; however the authors would tend to discourage excessive guessing.

The authors would like to extend their thanks to all those at the University of Manchester and elsewhere who aided their revision and helped to validate the content of these texts.

It only remains for the authors to wish you every success in your examination.

J. G. M. McDiarmid
C. A. Stone
December 1994

Recommended texts

Neville Wolff: *Cell Tissue and Disease,* 3rd Edition, Baillière Tindall, 1995.
  A good foundation for general pathology – better read before W+I.

Robbins, Cotran and Kumar: *A Pocket Companion to Robbins Pathologic Basis of Disease*, W. B. Saunders, 1990.
  Probably the most concise and compact book ever written, very good for systemic pathology revision.

J. B. Walter and M. S. Israel: *General Pathology*, Churchill Livingstone, 1994.
  Good reference text for systemic pathology.

1 INFLAMMATION AND THE IMMUNE SYSTEM

1 Human T cells
   A Have a lifespan of 5–10 years
   B Can neutralize bacterial toxins
   C Form immunoglobulins which drain into lymphatics
   D Release interferons which block viral mRNA transcription
   E Are able to bind free antigen in solution

2 Lymph
   A Has a high concentration of lymphocytes
   B Drain into venous blood
   C Has a higher protein concentration than plasma
   D Clots on standing
   E In the thoracic duct is 'milky' after a meal

3 Neutrophils
   A Form approximately 60% of the total white blood cells
   B Have a half-life of about one week
   C Move in and out of the bloodstream by diapedesis
   D Respond to chemotaxins
   E Form the superoxide anion

4 Macrophages
   A Are derived from megakaryocytes
   B Are chemotactic
   C Secrete interleukins
   D Act as antigen presentors
   E Have a half-life of about three days

5 Platelets
   A Are anuclear
   B Are stored in the spleen
   C Aggregate in response to prostacyclin
   D Form Von Willebrand's factor
   E Numbers are low in thrombasthenic purpura

6 IgGs
   A Form the majority of immunoglobulins
   B Are efficient opsonins
   C Of maternal origin are found in neonates
   D Are found on all B cells
   E Are formed against ABO blood antigens

INFLAMMATION – *Questions*

7 IgA
   - A Is abundant in sweat
   - B Of maternal origin is found in neonates
   - C Is active against both bacteria and viruses
   - D Forms dimers outside the plasma cells
   - E Is decreased in ataxia telangectasia

8 IgM
   - A Has a molecular weight around 900,000
   - B Is a weak complement fixator
   - C Forms the first post-immunization response
   - D Forms anti-rhesus antibodies
   - E Is implicated in the pathogenesis of rheumatoid arthritis

9 IgE
   - A Fab sites bind to mast cells
   - B Has binding sites for eosinophils
   - C Concentrations are genetically predetermined
   - D Is active against protozoa
   - E Is active against tubercle bacilli

10 Regarding complement
   - A It may be activated by toxoids
   - B Classically, is activated by Clq binding to Fab of IgM
   - C Pathways converge after C5 activation
   - D C5a is chemotactic
   - E C5a causes histamine release

11 Thymus independent antigens
   - A Trigger a T cell response in athymic people
   - B Are monomers
   - C Include pneumococcal polysaccharide
   - D Produce large numbers of memory cells
   - E Tolerance to these is readily induced

12 The following responses may occur in minutes rather than days
   - A Complement opsonization
   - B Phagocytosis
   - C Macrophage activation
   - D Proliferation of natural killer cells
   - E Transplant rejection

13 HIV is associated with
   - A Increased size of lymph nodes
   - B Increased susceptibility to tetanus
   - C Benign neoplasms of small skin blood vessels
   - D Increased numbers of T supressor cells
   - E Diarrhoea

INFLAMMATION — *Questions*

14 The autoimmune diseases include
   A Phacolytic opthalmitis
   B NIDDM
   C Rheumatic fever
   D Goodpasture's syndrome
   E Idiopathic thrombocytopenic purpura

15 Hypersensitivity
   A Anaphylaxis is known as type I hypersensitivity
   B May occur on first exposure to antigen
   C Steroids stabilize mast cell membranes
   D Releases preformed contents of mast cells
   E May cause vomiting and diarrhoea

16 Immune complex mediated hypersensitivity
   A Is known as type II hypersensitivity
   B Is implicated in Maple bark strippers disease
   C Is implicated in rheumatoid arthritis
   D Complexes form locally with antigenic excess
   E Activates complement

17 Cell mediated hypersensitivity may be seen in
   A Tuberculosis
   B Smallpox
   C Candidiasis
   D Organ rejection
   E Contact dermatitis

18 Type II hypersensitivity
   A Usually involves IgA
   B Cell lysis is usually complement induced
   C Is the type of sensitivity seen in transfusion reactions
   D Is responsible for serum sickness
   E May produce graft rejection

19 The following decrease the movement of inflammatory exudate into the extravascular compartment
   A Hypertension
   B Potassium
   C Piriton (chlorpheniramine)
   D Steroids
   E Lymphadenopathy

20 The following cause arteriolar dilatation and increased vascular permeability
   A Histamine
   B 5-HT
   C Heparin
   D SRSA (slow reacting substance of anaphylaxis)
   E Leukotrienes

INFLAMMATION – Questions

21 The following cause increased arteriolodilatation and increased vascular permeability
- A Bradykinin
- B PGI2
- C Potassium
- D C5a
- E Cortisol

22 Neutrophils
- A Have segmented nuclei within granular cytoplasm
- B Obtain energy via oxidative phosphorylation
- C Decrease their negative surface charge in response to chemotaxins
- D Weigh less than erythrocytes
- E Respond to chemokinesins

23 Chemotaxins
- A Act on the nuclear membrane of phagocytes
- B Are augmented by cAMP
- C Are inhibited by corticosteroids
- D Are activated by herpes simplex
- E Include denatured proteins

24 Macrophages secrete
- A Lymphokines
- B Endogenous pyrogen
- C Interferon
- D Hypochlorous acid
- E Histamine

25 The end result of acute inflammation may be
- A Resolution
- B Organization
- C Scarring
- D Tissue destruction
- E Regeneration

26 Resolution of acute inflammation
- A Tissue destruction may have occurred
- B Complete return to the pre-inflammatory state
- C Results when exudate persists
- D May occur in pneumonia
- E May result in decreased tissue function

27 Regeneration after acute inflammation
- A Implies no tissue destruction
- B Occurs to epithelial cells
- C Occurs in hepatic parenchyma
- D Occurs in cardiac muscle
- E Results in reduced function

INFLAMMATION — Questions

28 In healing by primary intention
   A Thrombus formation must first occur
   B Epidermal migration occurs on the second day
   C Epidermal mitosis increases almost immediately
   D Epidermal cells grow over surface clot
   E Epidermal migration occurs along suture tracks

29 In healing by primary intention
   A Epidermal growth is facilitated by chalones
   B Macrophages are necessary
   C Fibroblasts are the first inflammatory cells recruited
   D Small canalized capillaries grow into the wound area
   E The final stage is wound contraction

30 The following inhibit wound healing
   A Hyperascorbosis
   B Zinc
   C Keloid formation
   D Bone marrow irradiation
   E Wound irradiation

31 In repair of bone
   A Osteoblasts lay down new lamellar bone early
   B Piezoelectric forces aid bone remodelling
   C Osteoblasts are important
   D Hypervitaminosis D delays healing
   E Granulation tissue extends into marrow cavity

32 In granulomatous inflammation, epithelioid cells
   A Are a reaction to toxic, non-degradable matter
   B Consist of rounded cells in close contact
   C Are aggregated macrophages and plasma cells
   D Are rich in secretory granules
   E Have high phagocytic action

33 Epithelioid granulomata
   A May develop to form Langerhans giant cells
   B Nuclei enter mitosis in random manner
   C Polykaryon life-span exceeds that of a macrophage
   D Are low turnover type in response to silica
   E Persist until the irritant is cleared

34 Sarcoid
   A Is an epithelioid granuloma with central necrosis
   B May be found in any tissue
   C May be diagnosed serologically
   D May exhibit Ig light chains
   E Is thought to be virally transmitted

Inflammation — Questions

35 Dexon
 - A Is a synthetic long-chain carbohydrate
 - B Is absorbable
 - C Retains half its tensile strength in 50 days
 - D Is more rapidly absorbed than Vicryl
 - E Is more irritant than catgut

36 Regarding non-absorbable sutures
 - A Silk is a multifilament suture
 - B Less tissue reaction is caused if monofilament sutures are used
 - C Nylon sutures are well tolerated
 - D Nylon knots easily
 - E 6/0 Ethilon is stronger than 3/0

INFLAMMATION — Answers

1 A = True B = False C = False D = True E = False

B cell products, immunoglobulins, are able to neutralize bacterial toxins and bind free antigen in solution. T cells do not manufacture immunoglobulins.

2 A = True B = True C = False D = True E = True

Lymphocytes enter the circulation by draining via the lymphatics into the venous system. It contains less protein than plasma, though does contain enough clotting factors to allow it to clot *in vitro*. The lymphatics transport fats absorbed from the small intestine, accounting for its 'milky' appearance after a meal.

3 A = True B = False C = True D = True E = True

Neutrophils make up 40–70% of the white cell population and have a half-life of about 6 h. They diapedese in and out of the bloodstream, using it as a means of transport to accumulate at sites of acute inflammation in response to chemotaxins. Once at these sites they phagocytose inflammatory proteins and debris. The phagosomes so formed fuse with lysosomes whose contents include the superoxide anion, hydrogen peroxide and hypochlorous acid.

4 A = False B = True C = True D = True E = False

Platelets are derived from megakaryocytes. Macrophages both respond to chemotaxins (leaving the circulation as monocytes) and secrete them, e.g. interleukin 1, stimulating T helper cells. They can act as antigen presenting cells and have a half-life of about three months.

5 A = True B = True C = False D = False E = False

Twenty-five percent of platelets are stored in the spleen. Von Willebrand's factor is produced by platelets and endothelial cells and facilitate platelet adherence at injury sites. Prostacyclin (PGI2) inhibits platelet aggregation whereas thromboxanes (TX A2) stimulate it. Thrombasthenic purpura occurs when circulating platelets are abnormal.

6 A = True B = True C = True D = False E = False

Seventy-five percent of immunoglobulins are IgG. They fix complement and are used in opsonization of bacteria. They form monomers, so easily cross the placenta. IgM antibodies are found on all B cells and are those formed against ABO blood antigens.

7 A = True B = True C = True D = False E = True

IgA antibodies are abundant in secretions, tears, bile, milk and sweat. They coat bacteria and viruses to prevent adherence to mucosal surfaces. They are formed as dimers, with a joining 'J chain' within the plasma cell.

8 A = True B = False C = True D = False E = False

IgM is pentameric, having 5 ab binding sites with which to fix complement. They are responsible for the 'first wave' response to immunization. IgG antibodies are active against Rhesus antigens and to unknown antigens within the synovium and fluid in rheumatoid arthritis.

INFLAMMATION – Answers

9 **A** = False   **B** = False   **C** = True   **D** = True   **E** = False

IgE antibodies bind via Fc receptors to mast cells and basophils. Bound mast cells discharge histamine, leukotrienes and eosinophil chemotactic factor when the appropriate antigen binds to the Fab portion. The response is greater in atopic people, who are thought to produce large amounts of IgE. Immunological response to TB is via T cells.

10 **A** = False   **B** = False   **C** = False   **D** = True   **E** = False

The alternative pathway (activated by endotoxins) and classical pathway (by Clq binding to the Fc portion of IgG or IgM) converge after C3 activation. C3a and C5a are chemotactic, C3a also causes histamine release from mast cells, and C3b is an opsonin.

11 **A** = False   **B** = False   **C** = True   **D** = False   **E** = True

Thymus independent antigens trigger B cell responses in the absence of T cells. They are all polymers, for example pneumoccocal polysaccharide and dextran. The response is atypical in that few memory cells are produced, and tolerance is readily induced.

12 **A** = True   **B** = True   **C** = True   **D** = False   **E** = True

B and T cell responses take days to come into effect. However hyperacute transplant rejection occurs by way of preformed antibodies as a result of ABO incompatibility.

13 **A** = True   **B** = False   **C** = False   **D** = True   **E** = True

Tetanus is not an opportunistic infection and is not more likely in HIV patients. Kaposi's sarcoma is a malignant neoplasm of small skin blood vessels.

14 **A** = False   **B** = False   **C** = True   **D** = True   **E** = True

Phacogenic opthalmitis and IDDM are not thought to be autoimmune diseases.

15 **A** = True   **B** = False   **C** = False   **D** = True   **E** = True

Being immunologically mediated, hypersensitivity reactions do not occur on first exposure to antigen. The general steroid immunosuppressive qualities, and sodium chromoglycate act by stabilization of mast cell membranes, hence decreasing degranulation of preformed histamine, 5-HT, heparin, etc. Gastrointestinal disturbances such as pain, vomiting and diarrhoea may be related to food allergies.

16 **A** = False   **B** = True   **C** = True   **D** = False   **E** = True

This is type III hypersensitivity. Immune complexes are formed as a reaction to foreign proteins (e.g. spores of *Cryptostroma* in Maple bark strippers disease) or endogenous antigen (e.g. rheumatoid factor). They may form locally in situations of antibody excess or systematically in antigen excess. Damage is primarily caused by complement activation causing inflammation.

17 **A** = True   **B** = True   **C** = True   **D** = True   **E** = True

Type IV or cell mediated hypersensitivity is the principal pattern of response to *Mycobacterium tuberculosis*, fungi, protozoa, smallpox, and parasites as well as contact skin dermatitis and organ rejection. It is mediated by CD4+ T helper cells

INFLAMMATION — *Answers*

which secrete specific cytokines when activated by processed antigen presented in association with the MHC class II antigens. The secreted cytokines act by activation and recruitment of monocytes and macrophages.

18 A = False B = True C = True D = False E = True

Type II hypersensitivity is mediated by Igm or IgG antibodies directed at surface antigens. There are two main subtypes:
(1) Complement mediated cytotoxicity; in which IgG or IgM antibodies react with antigen to provoke complement activation and hence cell lysis. This is seen in transfusion reactions and erythroblastosis foetalis.
(2) Antibody dependent cell mediated cytotoxicity (ADCC): in which IgG antibody in combination with cell surface antigen is lysed by a non-sensitized cell with an Fc receptor such as monocytes, eosinophils and killer cells. This type of hypersensitivity may play a role in graft rejection. Serum sickness is an example of a type III immune complex mediated reaction.

19 A = False B = False C = True D = True E = True

Movement of exudate from intravascular to extravascular compartments is proportional to: (i) hydrostatic pressure difference, (ii) permeability of the endothelium and (iii) osmotic pressure difference between these components. Potassium accumulation causes precapillary dilatation causing increased hydrostatic pressure. Piriton is an antihistamine and steroids are generally anti-inflammatory, both reduce capillary permeability. Lymphadenopathy decreases afferent lymph flow, so increasing extravascular hydrostatic pressure.

20 A = True B = True C = False D = False E = False

Heparin is a cohabitor of mast cells and is not vasoactive. SRSA and leukotrienes cause sustained smooth muscle contraction, and are constrictor in nature.

21 A = True B = True C = False D = False E = False

Potassium causes arteriolar dilatation only and C5a complement increases permeability only. Cortisol, being a steroid, inhibits phospholipase A2 conversion to arachidonic acid and its prostaglandin metabolites, damping down the whole inflammatory process.

22 A = True B = False C = True D = False E = True

The granular cytoplasm stains densely with Romanowsky dyes, and neutrophils use glucose as their energy source. Chemotaxins decrease negative cell charge, so facilitating margination to the negative charged endothelium. The fact that they are heavier than erythrocytes is also thought to facilitate margination. Chemokinesins generally increase activity of phagocytic cells.

23 A = False B = False C = True D = False E = True

Acting at the plasma membrane, chemotaxins increase amounts of intracellular cGMP, promoting microtubule activity and directed movement. Steroids decrease amounts of prostaglandins which themselves increase cGMP. Some viruses, including herpes simplex, depress neutrophil movement. Chemotaxins include haemoglobin and albumin.

10 INFLAMMATION – *Answers*

24 A = False   B = True   C = True   D = True   E = False

Lymphokines from T lymphocytes, act on macrophages. Interferons give short-term protection against viruses. Histamine is secreted by mast cells.

25 A = True   B = False   C = True   D = False   E = True

With no tissue destruction, demolishing the inflammatory exudate results in resolution to the normal structure; persistent exudate progresses to organization then scarring. With destruction of tissues with non-dividing cells, scarring is the only outcome, whereas in other tissues providing an intact framework regeneration to the normal structure may occur.

26 A = False   B = True   C = False   D = True   E = True

Acute inflammation with no tissue destruction may result in resolution to the pre-inflammatory state once the exudate has been demolished. This occurs, for example, in lobar pneumonia.

27 A = False   B = True   C = True   D = False   E = False

Regeneration results if tissue destruction has occurred in labile (e.g. epithelial) or stable (e.g. parenchymous) cells so long as the cellular framework is intact. If the framework is destroyed, or the cells are permanent (e.g. cardiac muscle) then organization results in scarring.

28 A = False   B = False   C = False   D = False   E = True

The first step is formation of a fibrin-rich clot, followed by epithelial migration which begins after a few hours. Increased production of epithelial cells begins after 12 h to allow continued migration under the clot and along suture tracks.

29 A = False   B = True   C = False   D = False   E = False

The chalone hypothesis suggests that all epithelial cells produce chalones which inhibit their own reproduction. A cut epithelial surface secretes less chalones, so facilitating synthesis of more epithelial cells for migration. Macrophages are the first inflammatory cells present, fibroblasts being recruited after four or five days. Non-canalized capillary buds grow into the area and are only later canalized. Wound contraction occurs only in secondary intention healing.

30 A = False   B = False   C = False   D = False   E = True

Ascorbic acid (vitamin C) is necessary for, and zinc aids, wound healing. Keloid scarring is a result of excessive collagenation of a scar, causing it to grow outside its original boundary.

31 A = False   B = True   C = True   D = False   E = True

Osteoblasts lay down woven osteoid (uncalcified bone) initially. Piezoelectric forces and osteoclasts aid bone remodelling. Vitamin D deficiency causes bone failure of bone mineralization and would delay healing.

INFLAMMATION — *Answers*

32 A = False B = False C = False D = True E = False

Epithelioid granulomata occur due to lack of specific recognition by the immune system of persisting, non-toxic material. They consist of aggregations of elongated macrophages which are differentiated towards the secretory, rather than phagocytic, end of the macrophage activity spectrum.

33 A = True B = False C = False D = False E = True

Langerhans giant cells may develop from foreign body giant cells, being a more (secretory) specialized form of epithelioid granuloma. Individual nuclei enter mitosis synchronously to facilitate genetic pooling within the granuloma, though this results in polyploidy and reduced life-span. Silica is highly injurious to cells, so high turnover granulomata occur to maintain cell numbers until the irritant is cleared.

34 A = False B = True C = False D = False E = False

Sarcoidosis is characterized by well-formed epithelioid granulomata without central necrosis, and may be found in any organ or tissue. It is diagnosed by biopsy, and may exhibit Schaumann bodies and asteroid bodies but not Ig chains, which may be found in amyloidosis. It has been suggested that transmission may occur via scabies infestation.

35 A = True B = True C = False D = True E = False

Vicryl is absorbed more slowly than Dexon, and retains 50% of its tensile strength at 50 days. Catgut is a very irritant suture material, causing a marked inflammatory reaction.

36 A = True B = True C = True D = False E = False

All natural fibres (linen, cotton, silk) are multifilament, but tie easily. Monofilament suture material causes less tissue reaction and is less likely to harbour bacteria. All types of plastic material are well tolerated (propylene, polyesters, nylon) though nylon is better than most. The main disadvantage of nylon is slipping when knot tying. Sizes used in common practice range from 10/0 (for microvascular work) to 2/0 for muscle suturing.

2 THE PATHOLOGY OF SHOCK

1. Class I haemorrhage (loss of up to 15% blood volume)
   - A Produces a marked tachycardia as a primary response
   - B Results in a prolonged capillary refill time
   - C Is compensated for within 24 h without i.v. fluid resuscitation
   - D Requires fluid resuscitation with colloid but not blood
   - E Significantly compromises organ perfusion

2. Class II haemorrhage (loss of 15–20% blood volume)
   - A Produces an early tachycardia and increase in pulse pressure
   - B Requires crystalloid resuscitation
   - C Causes tachypnoea
   - D Commonly results in significant depression of consciousness
   - E Markedly decreases urine output

3. Class III haemorrhage (loss of 30–40% blood volume)
   - A Consistently causes systolic pressure to fall
   - B Requires resuscitation with crystalloid and blood
   - C Usually responds to an initial fluid bolus
   - D Central pulses may not be palpable
   - E Results in loss of consciousness

4. Class IV haemorrhage (loss of over 40% blood volume)
   - A Produces virtual anuria
   - B Is an indication for vasopressor therapy
   - C Resuscitation is by fully cross-matched blood alone
   - D Central venous access should be established routinely
   - E An urgent surgical referral should be considered

5. Early neural compensatory mechanisms during haemorrhagic shock include
   - A Fall in baroreceptor discharge
   - B Fall in chemoreceptor discharge
   - C Widespread active vasoconstriction
   - D Constriction of splanchnic vasculature
   - E Catecholamine release via adrenal medullary pre-ganglionic sympathetic neurones

6. The hormonal response to acute blood loss includes
   - A A reduction in ADH secretion
   - B Increased secretion of renin
   - C Increased secretion of growth hormone
   - D Increased secretion of hypothalamic CRH
   - E Increased secretion of insulin

7. The following occur at the cellular level during the metabolic ebb phase
   - A A decrease in red cell 2,3-dpg
   - B Decreased protein catabolism
   - C Increased peripheral glucose uptake
   - D Increased O_2 consumption
   - E Increased FFA utilization

14 THE PATHOLOGY OF SHOCK – *Questions*

8 Fluid and electrolyte changes in the first two days of shock include
   A Positive nitrogen balance
   B Positive water balance
   C Negative sodium balance
   D Expansion of plasma volume by 'autotransfusion'
   E Reduction in urine osmolality

9 Prolonged ischaemic hypoxia may typically cause
   A Pulmonary hyaline membrane formation
   B Centrilobular (zone 3) hepatocyte necrosis
   C Acute tubular necrosis
   D Subendocardial haemorrhage
   E Sheehan's syndrome

10 The following occur in advanced shock
   A A reduction in capillary permeability
   B Loss of arteriolar constriction whilst venoconstriction is maintained
   C Release of tissue thromboplastin
   D Release of a pancreatic myocardial depressant factor
   E Failure of cerebral autoregulation when arterial pressure reaches 80 mmHg

11 Cardiogenic shock
   A Requires rapid i.v. fluid resuscitation
   B Results in an increase in pulmonary artery wedge pressure
   C Complicates infarction of less than 10% of myocardium
   D Is a recognized sequel to cardiac surgery
   E Generally has a good prognosis

12 Septic shock
   A Is most commonly associated with Gram negative cocci
   B Cardiac output increases in early stages
   C Is mediated by activation of kinins
   D May have a fungal or viral cause in the immunosuppressed
   E Antibiotic therapy should await sensitivity results

13 Endotoxin
   A Is a lipopolysaccharide secreted by Gram negative bacteria
   B Has a direct negative inotropic effect on the heart
   C Causes activation of complement via the classical pathway
   D Causes activation of the clotting cascade via the intrinsic pathway
   E May cause Waterhouse–Freidrichsen syndrome

14 Anaphylactic shock
   A Is due to a widespread type IV hypersensitivity reaction
   B Is mediated mainly by IgM–Ag complexes
   C Total peripheral vascular resistance increases
   D Requires intravenous fluid resuscitation and adrenaline
   E May occur with an incompatible blood transfusion

THE PATHOLOGY OF SHOCK — *Questions*

15 In spinal shock
    A The patient is hypotensive, pale and sweaty
    B The bladder fills and empties reflexly
    C Tendon jerks exhibit hyperreflexia
    D Respiratory effort may be maintained with cervical injuries below C4
    E Sacral sparing is a good prognostic indicator

16 THE PATHOLOGY OF SHOCK – *Answers*

1   **A** = False   **B** = False   **C** = True   **D** = False   **E** = False

Class I haemorrhage (750 ml from a blood volume of 5 litres) produces no clinical signs apart from slight tachycardia in an otherwise healthy adult. Blood donation represents a reduction of this order in circulating blood volume.

2   **A** = False   **B** = True   **C** = True   **D** = False   **E** = False

Class II haemorrhage (750–1500 ml) results in an increase in diastolic pressure mediated by circulating catecholamines, but systolic pressure is relatively unaffected, hence pulse pressure drops. Tachycardia, tachypnoea, mild mental state changes and a slight drop in urine output are also features.

3   **A** = True   **B** = True   **C** = True   **D** = False   **E** = False

Hypotension occurs consistently only when over 1500–2000 ml of circulating blood volume are lost. Primary resuscitation is by crystalloid and by blood when available. Although most patients in this group respond to an initial fluid bolus, this is often unsustained. Loss of central pulses and of consciousness occurs when over 50% of circulating volume is lost.

4   **A** = True   **B** = False   **C** = False   **D** = False   **E** = False

Vasopressor agents are not used routinely in the management of shock except in the arrest situation. In class IV exsanguinating haemorrhage group specific or even O^- blood should be infused early via large bore cannulae sited in peripheral veins (cutdown if necessary). CVP lines may be useful in monitoring volumetric status in later stages of the resuscitation. Surgical involvement is mandatory in the resuscitation of the shocked patient and at 40% blood loss immediate surgical intervention is indicated.

5   **A** = True   **B** = False   **C** = True   **D** = True   **E** = True

Afferents from baroreceptors in the carotid sinus and aortic arch project via the IXth and Xth cranial nerves to the nucleus of the tractus solitarius in the medulla. Excitatory neurones relay to the cardioinhibitory centre, and inhibitory neurones to the vasomotor centre. Arterial hypotension decreases baroreceptor discharge, reducing cardiac inhibition and causing tachycardia, and increasing vasomotor activity and hence peripheral resistance. Chemoreceptors, stimulated by stagnant hypoxia in the aortic and carotid bodies, produce tachypnoea via the respiratory centre and vasoconstriction via the vasomotor centre. Although bradycardia is also an effect, this is overridden by catecholamine release and sympathetic tone.

6   **A** = False   **B** = True   **C** = True   **D** = True   **E** = False

Release of ADH from the posterior pituitary is increased following stimulation of low pressure receptors in the atria, great veins and pulmonary circulation, and also in response to angiotensin II and hypothalamic osmoreceptor stimulation. ADH promotes water reabsorption at the collecting ducts which expands plasma volume. Secretion of renin by juxtaglomerular cells acting as 'renal baroreceptors' increases as afferent arteriolar pressure falls, and in response to a fall in macula densa Na^+ and Cl^- transport at the distal convoluted tubule. Prostaglandins and sympathetic

THE PATHOLOGY OF SHOCK — Answers

activity also increase secretion. Renin converts circulating hepatic angiotensinogen to angiotensin I, the substrate for endothelial converting enzyme in production of angiotensin II. This is a potent vasoconstrictor, facilitates release of aldosterone and ADH, and exerts a dipsogenic effect on the subfornical organ.

An increase in ACTH secondary to CRH secretion stimulates secretion of glucocorticoids and aldosterone. Growth hormone is valuable for its diabetogenic effects, increasing glucose delivery to the brain.

7 A = False B = False C = False D = False E = True

Red cell 2,3-dpg increases and shifts the HbO_2 dissociation curve to the left. Glucocorticoids encourage protein catabolism in muscle to provide amino acids for hepatic gluconeogenesis. FFA synthesis by hormone sensitive lipase is stimulated by catecholamines, glucagon, ACTH, LH, TSH and 5-HT via a cAMP second messenger. Glucocorticoids, GH and thyroxine increase enzyme activity directly but at a slower rate. FFAs provide an alternative energy substrate to glucose. Oxygen consumption is decreased peripherally and metabolism moves towards anaerobic glycolysis which results in the lactic acidosis associated with hypovolaemic shock.

8 A = False B = True C = False D = True E = False

Protein catabolism leads to a negative nitrogen balance. Sodium and water are conserved by the kidney under the influence of aldosterone and potassium is lost. Urine volume falls and its osmolality rises. Capillary hydrostatic pressure falls and interstitial fluid moves into vessels, expanding plasma volume but causing intracellular dehydration.

9 A = True B = True C = True D = True E = True

10 A = False B = True C = True D = True E = False

Hypoxic damage to endothelium causes release of lysosomal enzymes and activation of inflammatory mediators including kinins and prostaglandins. Capillary permeability rises and protein leaks out of vessels, exacerbating intravascular volume depletion. The consequent rise in blood viscosity leads to sludging of red cells. Tissue thromboplastin is released activating factor X via the extrinsic pathway and microvascular thrombosis ensues. Myocardial ischaemia develops as heart rate increases and blood volume falls. Contractility is also compromised with the release of a myocardial depressant factor from the pancreas. As cerebral perfusion pressure falls to below 50 mmHg, depression of brain stem function leads to loss of autonomic regulation of vasomotor tone and cardiorespiratory drive. Vasodilation and bradycardia perpetuate the vicious cycle.

11 A = False B = True C = False D = True E = False

Cardiogenic shock complicates an estimated 10% of myocardial infarcts, most of which are extensive, affecting at least 45% of myocardium. Pulmonary congestion develops with acute heart failure and fluid resuscitation should proceed with extreme caution. Tamponade from leaking vessels or acute valve failure are causes of cardiogenic shock following cardiac surgery. Mortality is of the order of 70%.

18 THE PATHOLOGY OF SHOCK – *Answers*

12 A = False   B = True   C = True   D = True   E = False

The commonest organisms associated with septic shock are the Gram negative bacilli: *E. coli*, *Proteus* and *Klebsiella*. *Pseudomonas septicaemia* complicates major burns and *Staphococcus aureus* is the organism of tampon-related 'toxic shock syndrome'. Broad spectrum antibiotic therapy should be commenced immediately after taking samples for bacteriology. Septic shock strictly refers to pus-forming organisms. Viruses and fungi do not fall into this category.

13 A = False   B = True   C = False   D = True   E = True

Endotoxin is a cellwall lipopolysaccharide constituent of Gram negative bacteria. It activates the C3 protein of the complement system directly via the alternative pathway. Acute adrenocortical necrosis and insufficiency induced by a meningococcal endotoxin is known as the Waterhouse–Freidrichsen syndrome.

14 A = False   B = False   C = False   D = True   E = False

Anaphylactic shock is due to a type I hypersensitivity reaction. Mast cells bearing antigen-specific IgE on their surface degranulate when exposed to allergen causing massive histamine release. Histamine dilates vessels and increases permeability, enabling fluid to leak out of the circulation. Hypotension, urticaria and bronchospasm are the main features. An anaphylactic-type reaction can also occur via a type III hypersensitivity response. Introduction of antigen to a sensitized individual in whom large amounts of IgG exist (Arthus reaction) results in activation of complement via the alternative pathway and the production of intermediates including C3a and C5a which stimulate mast cell degranulation. Transfusion reaction is an example of a type II reaction, activation of complement proceeding along the classical pathway.

15 A = False   B = False   C = False   D = True   E = True

Complete autonomic paralysis below the level of the lesion in spinal shock results in loss of sympathetic vasoconstrictor tone with dependent pooling of blood. Hypotension ensues but there is a lack of sweating, which itself can lead to thermoregulatory problems especially in children.

Although the positive chronotropic effect on the heart is also lost, withdrawal of vagal tone may achieve a compensatory tachycardia. Lesions above C3 are associated with a high mortality due to apnoea; below this level some respiratory effort may be maintained. However, as tidal volume is often reduced progressive carbon dioxide retention may develop requiring mechanical ventilation. Tendon reflexes are depressed during the period of spinal shock, although persistence of the anal reflex is a good prognostic indicator. The bladder lacks tone and dilates until upper motor neurone injury features supervene and the bladder fills and empties 'automatically'.

3 Cardiac, Vascular and Respiratory Pathology

1. With respect to arteries and atheroma
   A   Elevated levels of low density lipoprotein (LDL) increases the risk of atheroma
   B   Elevated levels of high density lipoprotein (HDL) reduces the risk of atheroma
   C   LDL carries 40% of the serum cholesterol
   D   Hypertension is not an independent risk factor for atheroma development
   E   Good control of diabetes is unrelated to outcome in atheroma

2. Regarding atheroma
   A   The plaque has a superficial fibrous cap containing smooth muscle cells
   B   The cellular zone contains smooth muscle cells and T lymphocytes
   C   Lipid laden 'foam' cells are classical features of the cellular zone
   D   The smooth muscle cells are mono- or oligoclonal
   E   Infantile fatty streaks are of unknown significance

3. The following are true
   A   Polyarteritis nodosa is more commonly a disease of young male adults
   B   Wegener's granulomatosis is lethal in 80% of untreated patients within one year
   C   Temporal artery biopsy in giant cell arteritis has good sensitivity
   D   In thrombangitis obliterans atherosclerotic lesions are unusual
   E   In systemic lupus erythematosis (SLE) with Raynaud's syndrome, cervical sympathectomy is particularly helpful

4. Regarding abdominal aortic aneurysms
   A   Intact abdominal aortic aneurysms (AAA) are often painful
   B   'Renal colic' in a woman over 60 years is more likely to be a leaking AAA
   C   80% of AAAs over 6 cm in length rupture within two years
   D   Left thoracotomy to allow early control of the descending aorta is beneficial in ruptured AAA
   E   Ischaemic colitis is a complication of AAA repair

5. The following are contra-indications for non-cardiac elective surgery
   A   Myocardial infarct within the past six months
   B   Aortic stenosis
   C   A diastolic blood pressure of 110 mmHg
   D   Congestive cardiac failure
   E   Hypokalaemia

6. In ischaemic heart disease
   A   Angina doubles the risk of perioperative myocardial infarct (MI)
   B   Vasospasm is the usual cause of myocardial infarct
   C   Nitrates work by coronary artery vasodilatation
   D   Left ventricular function is not predictive of perioperative myocardial infarct rate
   E   Upper abdominal surgery is high risk for perioperative myocardial infarct

20 CARDIAC, VASCULAR AND RESPIRATORY – *Questions*

7 Regarding congenital cardiac disorders
   A Patent ductus arteriosus has a female preponderance
   B Approximately 30% of congenital cardiac defects have an environmental origin
   C Hypertrophic osteopathy is not seen in congenital cardiac disease
   D In transposition of the great arteries, a patent ductus arteriosus is essential for survival
   E In atrial septal defect (ASD) ostium primum defects are more common

8 In rheumatic fever
   A Definitive diagnosis requires the presence of three of the five Jones major criteria
   B Erythema marginatum may be seen in 50% of the cases
   C Mitral valve involvement alone is uncommon
   D Fever is one of Jones' major criteria
   E It is classically preceded by infection with a Lancefield group B streptococcus

9 In asthma
   A Smooth muscle in the airways is hyperplastic
   B Purulent sputum is usually due to an infection
   C In an acute attack the forced expiratory flow rate (FEF) is reduced by 25–75%
   D Impaired ventilatory capacity is responsible for the pO_2 being reduced
   E A rising pCO_2 in asthma denotes decreased minute ventilation

10 In chronic obstructive pulmonary disease (COPD)
   A Emphysema produces permanent dilation of the airways distal to the terminal bronchioles with destruction of their walls
   B Patients with α-1-antitrypsin deficiency frequently develop centrilobular emphysema
   C A Reid index of less than 0.5 is histologically diagnostic of chronic bronchitis
   D The pO_2 will fall on exercise
   E A raised pCO_2 indicates a chronic hypoventilatory state

11 Radiotherapy is efficacious for the following primary neoplasms of the lungs
   A Small cell carcinoma
   B Adenocarcinoma
   C Bronchioloalveolar carcinoma
   D Epidermoid carcinoma
   E Large cell carcinoma

CARDIAC, VASCULAR AND RESPIRATORY — Questions

12 In pulmonary embolism the following are true
   A Hypoxaemia without CO_2 retention is uncommon
   B Obstruction of the pulmonary artery leads to decreased ventilation of the unperfused lung
   C Physiological dead space is increased
   D Pulmonary infarction is common
   E Pulmonary embolus is associated with a loud first heart sound

13 The following are true
   A Ipratopium bromide may cause bronchoconstriction
   B Salbutamol increases smooth muscle cyclic AMP
   C Aminophylline excess produces gastrointestinal symptoms before cardiac side effects
   D Disodium chromoglycate is effective in acute asthma
   E Methylxanthines cause diuresis

14 Compliance is increased in the following
   A Rheumatic valvular disease
   B Asthma
   C Interstitial fibrosis
   D Emphysema
   E Pulmonary oedema

15 The following may cause adult respiratory distress syndrome
   A Long bone fracture
   B Burns
   C Goodpasture's syndrome
   D Cardiopulmonary bypass
   E Pancreatitis

16 Regarding mechanical ventilation
   A Endotracheal tubes can be safely left in place for weeks
   B Intermittent positive pressure ventilation (IPPV) generally reduces cardiac output
   C 100% O_2 is appropriate throughout ventilation
   D Ileus is common
   E Pneumothorax is a recognized complication

22 CARDIAC, VASCULAR AND RESPIRATORY – *Answers*

1   **A** = True   **B** = True   **C** = False   **D** = False   **E** = False
LDL carries 70% of the serum cholesterol.

2   **A** = True   **B** = True   **C** = False   **D** = True   **E** = True
The theories of atheromatous plaque formation are: (i) intimal injury results in collagen exposure to which platelets adhere. The platelet derived growth factor (PDGF) produced by these platelets produces smooth muscle cell proliferation.
(ii) Neoplastic smooth muscle cells proliferate (monoclonally).
   A plaque contains three zones
(i)   Superficial fibrous cap – containing smooth muscle cells and dense fibrous tissue
(ii) Cellular – containing smooth muscle cells, macrophages and T lymphocytes
(iii) Necrotic central zone – containing cholesterol and lipid 'foam' cells.

3   **A** = True   **B** = True   **C** = False   **D** = True   **E** = False
In giant cell arteritis 40% of temporal artery biopsies are negative on examination and therefore the test is not very sensitive. Thrombangitis obliterans is a disease of young smokers and hence atherosclerotic plaques are unusual. The Raynaud's syndrome seen in patients with SLE is intractable and cervical sympathectomy provides temporary benefit only.

4   **A** = True   **B** = True   **C** = False   **D** = False   **E** = True
Fifty percent of patients with AAA have back pain or sciatica. Inflammatory AAA and expanding AAA also cause pain. Pain is an indication for operation. De Dombal's figures suggest B to be true. Half of AAA over 6 cm in length will rupture within two years. The transperitoneal approach is preferred and clamping distal to the renal arteries is ideal when circumstances allow. The inferior mesenteric artery (IMA) is inevitably sacrificed during repair and ischaemic colitis may result.

5   **A** = True   **B** = True   **C** = False   **D** = True   **E** = True
Surgery within six months of myocardial infarct (MI) increases the risk of reinfarct. Reinfarct rates are ~25% within six months and this drops to 5% thereafter; 70% of reinfarcts die. Aortic stenosis is a fixed output state. Any drop in vascular resistance produces a drop in blood pressure (BP) and lowers cerebral, coronary and renal perfusion. Hypertensive individuals have non-compliant vasculature with high resting sympathetic tone. Anaesthesia can lead to precipitous blood pressure drops. Despite this a diastolic BP up to 110 mmHg seems to have little effect on perioperative mortality. Congestive cardiac failure even when controlled has a high surgical mortality. Hypokalaemia interacts with digoxin, diuretics and hyperventilation to produce arrhythmias.

6   **A** = False   **B** = False   **C** = False   **D** = False   **E** = True
Angina increases infarct risk to 10–50 times that of a normal patient. Coronary artery stenosis secondary to atheroma is the normal cause of MI. Nitrates produce venodilatation and hence reduce cardiac preload and cardiac work. Left ventricular function is an important predictor of infarct potential, as is triple vessel disease. Chest, upper abdominal and surgery continuing for more than 3 h are all associated with a four-fold increase in MI rate.

CARDIAC, VASCULAR AND RESPIRATORY — *Answers*

7 A = True B = False C = False D = True E = False

Less than 1% of congenital cardiac defects are solely attributable to environmental origin (e.g. maternal rubella). Hypertrophic osteopathy and/or finger clubbing are commonly seen in congenital cardiac disease. Only 5% of ASDs are due to ostium primum defect.

8 A = False B = True C = False D = False E = False

Diagnoses of rheumatic fever requires the presence of two of the five major criteria. Mitral valve involvement alone is seen in 60–70% of cases. Classically an infection with a Lancefield group A streptococcus precedes the onset of rheumatic fever by one to five weeks.

9 A = False B = False C = True D = False E = True

In asthma smooth muscle is typically hypertrophied. Eosinophils tend to make sputum purulent in the absence of infection. In acute asthma all indices of expiratory rate are reduced. V/Q mismatching is responsible for the reduction in pO_2. pCO_2 is normally also reduced due to hyperventilation, and a rising pCO_2 denotes fatigue and a secondary reduction in ventilation rate and tidal volume: this is a sign of impending death and the need for ventilation.

10 A = True B = False C = True D = False E = False

Emphysema is anatomically defined as A. α-1-Antitrypsin deficiency leads to a panlobular pattern of emphysema. The Reid index is a histologically measured ratio of submucosal gland thickness to total mucosal and submucosal thickness; 0.5 is taken as diagnostic of COPD. On exercise the pO_2 may rise or fall. It will tend to fall in the presence of limited reserve of cardiac output and limited respiratory reserve. A raised pCO_2 may well indicate hypoventilation, but gives no indication of chronicity.

11 A = False B = False C = False D = True E = False

Small cell carcinoma is amenable to chemotherapy. In any tumour causing bone pain or superior vena cava obstruction radiotherapy may produce temporary respite.

12 A = False B = True C = True D = False E = False

Hypoxaemia without CO_2 retention is normal. V/Q mismatch is responsible for the former and increased ventilation for the latter. Obstruction of the pulmonary artery is a phenomenon of bronchoconstriction that is reversed by addition of CO_2 to inspired gas. Due to ventilation perfusion mismatch physiological dead space is increased. Pulmonary infarction is uncommon partially due to the protective effect of the bronchial arteries. A loud second heart sound due to pulmonary hypertension is heard in pulmonary embolism.

13 A = True B = True C = False D = False E = True

Ipratopium bromide is an anticholinergic drug but it may cause bronchoconstriction and administration of the first dose should be observed. Salbutamol and methylxanthines increase smooth muscle cyclic AMP and hence stabilize the smooth muscle. Chromoglycate stabilizes mast cells and is of use as prophylaxis for allergic asthma.

24 CARDIAC, VASCULAR AND RESPIRATORY – *Answers*

14 **A** = False   **B** = True   **C** = False   **D** = True   **E** = False

Compliance relates inversely to the 'stiffness' and elasticity of lung tissue. Fibrosis, oedema and chronic high pulmonary capillary pressure increase 'stiffness'. Emphysema destroys elasticity. The increase in compliance in asthma is due to obscure reasons, but tends to prove that it is a disease of obstructed expiration and not inspiration.

15 **A** = True   **B** = True   **C** = True   **D** = True   **E** = True

Adult respiratory distress syndrome follows increased pulmonary circulatory permeability. Theory states that white cell and platelet aggregates from any part of the body are trapped within the pulmonary capillary bed. This results in an acute inflammatory reaction within the capillary bed with release of serotonin, histamine, leukotrienes and kinins.

16 **A** = True   **B** = False   **C** = False   **D** = True   **E** = True

Cardiac output is generally stable during IPPV. Prolonged therapy with 100% O_2 may induce toxicity.

4 Gastrointestinal and Hepatobiliary Pathology

1 In achalasia
   A There is a lack of peristalsis
   B There is increased tone at the lower oesophageal sphincter
   C Approximately 5% of cases lead on to malignancy
   D There is a female preponderance
   E The myenteric plexus has hypertrophied

2 Regarding Mallory–Weiss syndrome
   A At endoscopy 30% of upper gastrointestinal bleeds are due to it
   B It has a mortality rate of 2%
   C Often involves multiple oesophageal tears
   D It is more common in alcoholics
   E Hiatus hernia is a risk factor

3 In pyloric stenosis
   A A succussion splash is rare
   B Hypochloraemia results
   C Hypokalaemia results
   D Aciduria results
   E Acidosis occurs

4 Regarding peptic ulcers
   A Less than 60% of duodenal ulcers are within 2 cm of the pylorus
   B Duodenal ulcer (DU) is associated with HLA B5
   C DU is more common in chronic renal failure
   D Gastrinoma tends to be malignant
   E Blood group A is a risk factor for DU

5 The following distinguish ulcerative colitis from Crohn's disease
   A Sacroileitis
   B Transmural inflammation
   C Pseudopolyps
   D Crypt abscesses
   E Granulomas

6 Regarding gallstones
   A Cholesterol stones are most common
   B There is a female preponderance
   C Diabetes mellitus increases the mortality from cholecystitis in individuals with gallstones
   D They are generally radio-opaque
   E Cystic fibrosis is a risk factor for their development

7 In carcinoid tumour

   A The appendix is the most common site of origin
   B Metastases are rarely present at time of diagnosis
   C Raised urinary serotonin is diagnostic
   D Doxorubicin is an effective agent for the treatment of carcinoid
   E Somatostatin slows tumour growth

8 Bowel lengths in adults

   A 1 m of small bowel has sufficient absorption capacity for survival
   B 1 m of distal ileum is required to avoid malabsorption
   C In short bowel, blind loop syndrome is more common
   D In short bowel, gastric hypersecretion is more common
   E Renal stones occur in up to 10% of patients with short bowel syndromes

9 The following pathologies are associated with the listed histological patterns in the liver

   A Gilbert's syndrome – centrilobular necrosis
   B Right heart failure – nutmeg liver – ischaemic centrilobular necrosis
   C Halothane toxicity – periportal necrosis
   D Eclampsia – midzone necrosis
   E Chronic persistent hepatitis – bridging necrosis

GASTROINTESTINAL PATHOLOGY — Answers

1   **A** = True   **B** = True   **C** = True   **D** = False   **E** = False

Achalasia is characterized by aperistalsis with raised lower oesophageal sphincter tone. Dysplastic mucosa is common and results in malignancy in approximately 5% of sufferers. There is a male preponderance and incidence peaks between the ages of 30–60. The myenteric plexus is atrophied and degenerated.

2   **A** = False   **B** = True   **C** = True   **D** = True   **E** = True

Five to ten percent of upper gastrointestinal bleeds which are endoscoped have Mallory–Weiss syndrome. Up to 10% may require surgery and a 2% mortality is quoted. Twenty-five percent have multiple tears of the oesophagus. Alcoholism is common and two-thirds of Mallory–Weiss tears occur in association with a hiatus hernia.

3   **A** = False   **B** = True   **C** = True   **D** = True   **E** = False

Succussion splash is present in nearly all advanced cases of pyloric stenosis. The vomiting resulting from pyloric stenosis causes loss of H^+, Cl^-, K^+, Na^+ and water leading to hypokalaemic hypochloraemic alkalosis. Renal response is through Na^+ preservation leading to further loss of H^+ and K^+ in the urine.

4   **A** = False   **B** = True   **C** = True   **D** = True   **E** = False

Ninety percent of DUs are within 2 cm of the pylorus. HLA B5 is a risk factor for DU, and it is more common in patients with chronic renal failure, chronic obstructive pulmonary disease and hyperparathyroidism. Sixty percent of gastrinomas in Zollinger–Ellison syndrome are malignant. Blood group A is a risk factor for gastric carcinoma. Blood group O is a risk factor for DU.

5   **A** = False   **B** = True   **C** = False   **D** = False   **E** = True

Crohn's disease has skip lesions, non-caseating granulomas and full thickness inflammation. Ulcerative colitis begins in the rectum and extends proximally in continuity, it shows pseudopolyps and dysplasia. Both have systemic symptoms associated with HLA B27; iritis, sacroileitis, ankylosing spondylitis and both show crypt abscesses.

6   **A** = False   **B** = True   **C** = True   **D** = False   **E** = True

Mixed stones are by far the most common, although cholesterol is a component in most. The male to female ratio is 1:2. Serious complications and death are more common in the elderly and those with diabetes mellitus. Ten percent are radio-opaque. The abnormal mucus in cystic fibrosis produces a nidus for stone formation.

7   **A** = True   **B** = False   **C** = False   **D** = False   **E** = False

The appendix, followed by the small bowel, is the commonest site for carcinoid development. Carcinoid from the appendix rarely metastasises, however 45% of carcinoid tumours have metastasized by time of diagnoses. Raised urinary 5-hydroxyindoleacetic acid is diagnostic. Doxorubicin produces only a 20% response rate and is not generally used. Somatostatin particularly helps diarrhoea but does not influence tumour growth.

8   **A** = False   **B** = False   **C** = True   **D** = True   **E** = True

Patients with 1 m of small bowel or less often require parenteral nutrition indefinitely. Resection of 1 m of terminal ileum leads to bile salt, cholesterol and vitamin B_{12} malabsorption. Blind loop syndrome is more common in individuals with short bowel syndrome possibly due to a shorter small bowel being easier to colonize. In malabsorption, fatty acids bind calcium leaving oxalate unbound (calcium oxalate is insoluble). Unbound oxalate is absorbed in colon and results in renal oxalate stones.

9   **A** = False   **B** = True   **C** = False   **D** = False   **E** = False

Gilbert's syndrome is one of glucuronidation impairment and is not associated with any morphological changes. Congestion and back pressure on hepatic veins leads to centrilobular necrosis. Halothane and yellow fever cause midzonal necrosis. Eclampsia and phosphorus poisoning cause periportal necrosis. Chronic persistent hepatitis results in periportal chronic inflammatory infiltrate and no necrosis.

5 Renal Pathology

1. Chronic renal failure (CRF) is associated with
   - A Hypercalcaemia
   - B Elevated parathyroid hormone levels
   - C Fibrosis of bone
   - D Polycythaemia
   - E Congestive cardiac failure

2. The following cause urinary tract infections in the normal adult
   - A *Cryptococcus*
   - B Vesicoureteric reflux
   - C Gram negative bacilli
   - D Analgesic nephropathy
   - E Urethral instrumentation

3. Renal cell carcinoma
   - A Affects the young
   - B Produces haematuria consistently
   - C May spread early to inferior vena cava
   - D Causes polycythaemia
   - E Malignant cells originate from cortical tubules

4. The following predispose to the formation of renal calculi
   - A Isolated hypercalciuria
   - B Prostatic hypertrophy
   - C Altered urinary pH
   - D Urease-splitting organisms
   - E Neurogenic bladder

5. Transitional cell bladder tumours are
   - A Frequently recurrent
   - B Less common than adenocarcinomas
   - C Cause haematuria
   - D Carcinomas more commonly than papillomas
   - E Invasive

6. Diabetes mellitus is associated with the following
   - A Diffuse and nodular glomerulosclerosis
   - B Benign nephrosclerosis and hypertension
   - C Nephrotic syndrome
   - D Acute glomerulonephritis
   - E Urinary tract infection

7. Acute renal failure is associated with
   - A Severe crush injury
   - B Casts in distal convoluted tubules
   - C Tubular necrosis invariably
   - D Polyuria
   - E Hyperkalaemia

8 The following types of renal damage may occur in benign hypertension
  A Nephron and cortical atrophy
  B Marked increase in renin levels
  C Hyaline arterial wall thickening
  D Chronic renal failure
  E Hyperplastic arteriosclerosis (onion skinning)

RENAL PATHOLOGY – *Answers*

1 **A** = False **B** = True **C** = True **D** = False **E** = True

In CRF impaired hydroxylation of hydroxyvitamin D_3 occurs, leading to impaired absorption of calcium from the bowel. Resultant hypocalcaemia stimulates parathyroid hyperplasia and compensatory secondary hyperparathyroidism. Renal osteodystrophy may occur in CRF and involves bone changes including excessive osteoclastic resorption and trabecular and marrow fibrosis. Erythropoietin production is reduced with worsening anaemia to compound the marrow dysfunction. The multiplicity of fluid and electrolyte disturbances of renal failure predispose to cardiac overload and oedema.

2 **A** = False **B** = True **C** = True **D** = False **E** = True

Atypical organisms such as *Candida* and *Cryptococcus* only cause infections in immunocompromised hosts. More than 85% of caustive organisms in the normal host are Gram negative bacilli. Reflux nephropathy, with its onset in childhood, is the main cause of urinary tract infections or on-going low-grade infection. However, some cases have sterile pyuria with a latent, insidious presentation. Analgesic nephritis may cause polyuria and pyuria, however the latter is usually sterile also.

3 **A** = False **B** = True **C** = True **D** = True **E** = True

These adenocarcinomas seldom occur below 40 years, sometimes arising from pre-existing cortical adenomas, with tumours over 3 cm arousing a high index of suspicion. They originate from renal tubular cells and microscopically contain a variety of cell types including clear, granulated and undifferentiated forms. Although haematuria occurs in 90% of cases, symptoms appear typically late, with breach of renal pelvis and capsule and direct macroscopic spread along the renal vein in 20% of cases. Haematogenous metastases to lung, bone and brain also occur relatively early. Clinical manifestation may be via a paraneoplasic syndrome, i.e not directly related to tumour spread or involvement, as is the case with polycythaemia.

4 **A** = False **B** = True **C** = True **D** = True **E** = True

Impairment of bladder emptying either through autonomic dysfunction or outflow obstruction, allows colonization of residual urine. Alteration of urinary pH, alters the solubility of salts which may form the constituents of stones including calcium, magnesium and uric acid. The former compose 75% of all stones and only 75% of these have a demonstrable metabolic abnormality. The organism *Proteus* efficiently converts urea into ammonia which lowers the acidity and hence causes the formation of stones.

5 **A** = True **B** = False **C** = True **D** = True **E** = False

Transitional cell tumours form the majority of epithelial bladder tumours, others being squamous and very rarely adenocarcinomas. Squamous tumours have a particular association with schistosomal infections, whilst adenocarcinomas are usually found at the bladder base where glandular tissues or urachal remnants lie. Transitional cell tumours form a spectrum of cellular atypia and usually papillary exophytic growth patterns, however they are all potentially invasive and therefore malignant (i.e. carcinomas). Higher grade lesions are solid and infiltrative. They are typically multiple or recurrent and the prognostically worse tumours typically cause painless haematuria.

RENAL PATHOLOGY – *Answers*

6   A = True   B = True   C = False   D = False   E = True

The pathogenesis of diabetic complications is dependent upon metabolic derangements. With hyperglycaemia, renal cells take up glucose freely and independently of insulin, and it is intracellular hyperglycaemia that stimulates and promotes increased osmotic activity with cellular swelling, but more importantly, the non-enzymatic glycosylation of vascular and tubular epithelial enzyme systems and basement membranes. This results in diffuse thickening of the basement membranes of renal glomerular capillaries and the consequent ischaemia causes glomerulosclerosis. Chronic renal failure and proteinuria are progressive, the former is a leading cause of death in diabetics but the latter seldom reaching the levels of nephrotic syndrome. Arteriosclerosis is widespread, not confined to kidneys and results in chronic hypertension. Glycosuria enhances urine as a culture medium and this in turn may be exacerbated by any autonomic nervous dysfunction of the bladder. Recurrent infections predispose to papillary inflammation and necrosis.

7   A = True   B = True   C = False   D = True   E = True

Acute renal failure and acute tubular necrosis are not synonymous, other causes of acute renal failure include vascular or urinary obstruction or glomerulonephritis which may spare tubular epithelium. However, ATN is apparent often with causative insults being ischaemic or nephrotoxic, in particular sepsis, burns or crush injury, the latter with its rhabdomyolysis and glomerular obstruction by myoglobin. Necrosis occurs in the proximal segments and cellular casts are found in relatively spared distal tubules and collecting ducts. Early on, failing tubular cells are unable to excrete potassium, but hypokalaemia and polyuria may dramatically ensue in the recovery stage.

8   A = True   B = False   C = True   D = False   E = False

Benign nephrosclerosis is a conglomerate term for the renal changes associated with benign hypertension. These include hyaline sclerosis of arterioles and fibroelastic hyperplasia of arteries. The vascular changes cause nephron atrophy and a decrease in cortical dimensions. Increased renin is a more important mechanism in conditions such as renal artery stenosis, vaculitides, malignant hypertension and tumours. Only 1–5% of cases of benign nephrosclerosis lead to chronic renal failure and the majority of these show a transient malignant hypertensive phase. This latter is pathognomonically associated with prolific arteriolar hyperplasia, sclerosis (onion-skin appearance on section of vessels) and necrosis of arterioles and hence glomeruli.

6 FRACTURE HEALING AND THE MUSCULOSKELETAL SYSTEM

1 The following are associated with excessive osteoclastic activity and bone resorption
   A Osteogenesis imperfecta
   B Osteopetrosis
   C Osteoporosis
   D Uncompensated osteomalacia
   E Hyperpathyroidism

2 The following commonly occur around the knee joint
   A Osteoid osteoma in the young
   B Osteosarcoma in the young
   C Chondrosarcoma
   D Enchondroma
   E Bursitis

3 The following impair the healing of fractures
   A Sequestrum
   B Fibroblast activation
   C Weightbearing
   D Avitaminosis
   E Osteoid formation

4 Ischaemic necrosis of bone is associated with the following
   A Femoral neck fractures
   B Tibial plateau fractures
   C Sickle cell crisis
   D Scaphoid fracture
   E Elbow dislocations

5 Osteoblastic skeletal metastases occur in carcinoma of the
   A Stomach
   B Prostate
   C Breast
   D Ovary
   E Malignant lymphoma

6 Secondary tumours of bone
   A Are more common than all primary malignant tumours together
   B Predispose to pathological fractures
   C All tumour emboli result in metastases
   D Occur most commonly in the spine
   E Spare intervertebral discs

7   Soft tissue sarcomas

    A   Are vascular with early haematogenous dissemination
    B   Are malignant, ectodermal, connective tissue tumours
    C   Occur frequently in the young
    D   More differentiated types have worse prognosis
    E   All arise from pre-existing benign tumours

8   Paget's disease of bone is associated with the following

    A   Increased osteoclastic activity
    B   Increased osteoblastic activity
    C   Increased cardiac output
    D   Malignant change
    E   Elevated serum alkaline phosphatase

FRACTURE HEALING – *Answers*

1 **A** = False **B** = False **C** = True **D** = False **E** = True

Osteogenesis imperfecta or 'brittle bones' is a genetically abnormal synthesis of type I collagen. Osteopenia results due to decreased matrix production, with a predisposition to fracture. Osteopetrosis or marble bones is bone overgrowth, with sclerosis, cortical thickening and even encroachment on the medullary cavity. Herediterally, osteoclast function is defective. Osteoporosis, a reduction of fully mineralized matrix, results from not only a decrease in osteoblast numbers but also an increase in osteoclastic resorption. Osteomalacia from whatever cause is a metabolic failure to fully mineralize bone with an excess of unmineralized matrix when, as often, it is associated with a low serum calcium, secondary hyperparathyroidism results. Excess parathyroid hormone mobilizes mineral from bone via increased osteclastic resorption.

2 **A** = True **B** = True **C** = True **D** = False **E** = True

Ninety percent of osteoid osteomas occur under the age of 25 years, and although benign, cause pain in the femur or tibia around the knee. The majority of osteosarcomas occur below 25 years in metaphyses of long bones, predominantly distal femur and proximal tibia. These primary cases arise *de novo* but there is also a peak incidence in an older age group on a background of existing pathology. These cases occur equally in incidence between long bones and flat bones. Enchondromas are benign, occurring singly or multiply, in phalanges of the hands most commonly, but also in ends of long bones. Bursitis (housemaid's knee) is common.

3 **A** = True **B** = False **C** = False **D** = True **E** = False

A sequestrum forms as a result of suppurative infection with cortical deprivation of its endosteal and periosteal vascular supply. The dead fragment of sequestrum, remains a nidus for infection. In the healing of fractures, haematoma organization and inflammatory cell infiltration occur concomitantly, fibroblasts are integral to this. The osteoid or osseous callus is later remodelled along lines of weightbearing stresses, although excess loading too early may impair healing.

4 **A** = True **B** = False **C** = True **D** = True **E** = True

Femoral head and scaphoid bones typically have a large distally based vascular supply and these may be partially jeopardized by subcapital neck of femur fractures and those of the waist of scaphoid. Arterial anastomoses around the knee and elbow joints are complex and rich, and fracture-dislocations require immediate and adequate alignment as arterial supply to structures distal to these points may become compromised. Sickle cells have rigid, non-deformable cell membranes and produce embolic vaso-occlusive crises with resultant painful ischaemic necrosis.

5 **A** = False **B** = True **C** = True **D** = False **E** = True

Many skeletal metastases destroy bone producing osteolytic lesions. Some malignant cell types evoke an osteoblastic response also with sclerotic lesions. They include prostatic carcinoma and occasionally breast secondaries and Hodgkin's disease. The others commonly metastasize to bone except ovarian carcinoma which tends to earlier direct involvement of other pelvic organs, lymphatic or transcoelomic spread.

FRACTURE HEALING – Answers

6 A = True B = True C = False D = True E = True

Bone metastases are present in up to one fifth of fatal malignant disease with preponderance to the vertebral column with not infrequently collapse of the bodies. The discs are typically spared until late in the disease as firstly, spinal arteries enter and feed the spinal column at the midpoints of the vertebrae first, and secondly that the discs are relatively avascular. Of course, not all haematogenous tumour emboli become metastases, requiring favourable local environment to seed and invade.

7 A = True B = False C = False D = False E = False

Sarcomas are malignancies of mesodermal origin, arising from any of the individual connective tissue types, the host tissue lending its name as prefix to the tumour type, e.g. fibrosarcoma, leiomyosarcoma. Undifferentiated types without a diagnostic stroma do occur and have a worse prognosis with early blood-borne dissemination. Although some arise from benign tumours most arise *de novo*. Soft tissue sarcomas are very rare tumours occurring most commonly in older individuals.

8 A = True B = True C = True D = True E = True

Increased blast and clast activity occur concomitantly, although earlier stages are dominated by bone resorption by numerous overlarge osteoclasts, sclerosis results latterly. New bone is laid down in a distinct mosaic pattern and is disorganized, poorly mineralized and soft. Spaces in between are occupied by fibrous tissue containing large vascular lacunae with high flow. Approximately 1% of cases show secondary sarcomatous change. Elevated alkaline phosphotase is a reflection of osteoblastic activity.

7 THE ENDOCRINE SYSTEM

1. The following are true regarding pituitary adenomas
   - A Most produce hormones, commonly thyroid-stimulating hormone
   - B May produce hyponatraemia
   - C Are not invasive
   - D May be associated with multiple endocrine neoplastic syndrome
   - E May produce hypopituitarism

2. Thyroid conditions showing follicular cell hypertrophy and hyperplasia include
   - A Hashimoto's thyroiditis
   - B Graves' disease
   - C Diffuse non-toxic goitre
   - D Adenoma
   - E Medullary carcinoma

3. Cushing's syndrome is associated with
   - A Pathologicial fractures
   - B Positive nitrogen balance
   - C Poor wound healing
   - D Hyperkalaemia
   - E Polyuria

4. Changes associated with primary hyperparathyroidism include
   - A Polyuria and nephrocalcinosis
   - B Hypokalaemia
   - C Peptic ulcer disease
   - D Dystrophic calcification
   - E Bone cysts and elevated alkaline phosphatase

5. Hormone-producing tumours
   - A All arise from endocrine tissue
   - B Feedback on normal endocrine tissue
   - C Are independent of control
   - D All normally secrete normal hormones
   - E Originate from embryonic ectoderm

6. The following produce endocrine effects
   - A Medullary carcinoma of thyroid
   - B Phaeochromocytoma
   - C Neuroblastoma
   - D Gastrinoma
   - E Small cell bronchial carcinoma

38 THE ENDOCRINE SYSTEM — Answers

1   **A** = False   **B** = False   **C** = True   **D** = True   **E** = True

Adenomas constitute 15% of all primary intracranial tumours; carcinomas at this site being rare. Of the former, 70% elaborate hormones, usually growth hormone, prolactin, ACTH or a mixture of the two, TSH and gonadotrophin production being rare. The remainder are non-functional but through direct growth, expand and may invade contiguous structures – compression of remaining normal gland producing hypopituitarism and pressure or invasion of posterior lobe to cause insufficient ADH with resulting diabetes insipidus. This will tend to elevate serum sodium to upper limits of normal excacerbated by any excess in ACTH and hence corisol production. MEN type I syndrome includes hyperplastic or tumourous pituitary, parathyroid, adnenal glands and pancreatic islet hyperplasia.

2   **A** = False   **B** = True   **C** = True   **D** = True   **E** = False

All the above conditions are goitrous but not all due to proliferation of host follicular elements. Autoimmune thyroiditis shows abundance of lymphoid and plasma cell infiltration, formation of germinal centres and a variable amount of fibrosis. Follicular cells involute and transform with diminished colloid. In Graves', stimulating and growth autoantibodies lead to hyperaemic, lymphocytic glandular enlargement, predominated by hyperplastic, tall follicular epithelium with papillary processes crowding progressively deficient colloid. Diffuse non-toxic goitrous glands react by hypertrophy of the thyroid in order to maintain a euthyroid state. Initial changes are of follicular epithelial hypertrophy with scant colloid. Later there are variable amounts of epithelial involution and colloid accumulation. Adenomas have isolated follicular proliferation. Medullary carcinoma is derived from parafollicular neuroendocrine calcitonin secreting cells.

3   **A** = True   **B** = False   **C** = True   **D** = False   **E** = True

Excess glucocorticoid action effects gluconeogenesis from protein and fat catabolism to cause hyperglycaemia, glycosuria and polyuria. This is exacerbated by impaired glucose tolerance and the effect of increased free water clearance by cortisol. Protein catabolism and reduced synthesis leads to osteoporosis and impairs wound healing, the latter abetted by disturbed lymphoid function and impaired response to infection. Nitrogen, from protein and amino acid conversion, is lost in urine. The mineralocorticoid effect of cortisol is weak unless in excess, when K^+ ions are lost in exchange for Na^+.

4   **A** = True   **B** = True   **C** = True   **D** = False   **E** = True

This accounts for one third of cases of hypercalcaemia. The primary problem is of excessive resorption and mobilization of calcium from bone, leaving rarification, cysts and subperiosteal erosions, most evident radiographically in the distal phalanges. Prolonged decalcification leads to secondary osteoblastic reaction, rich in alkaline phosphatase to cause its elevation. The majority of presenting features are due to high free ionized calcium. Metastatic calcification (deposition of calcium salts in extraosseous sites associated with hypercalcaemia) occurs rather than dystrophic calcification (calcification of non-viable or dying tissues with normal serum calcium), should the solubility be exceeded. Initially tubular epithelium has impaired response to ADH and latterly tubular calcification may also impair ability to concentrate urine. Calcium inhibits potassium reabsorption from tubular lumen and stimulates gastrin secretion from gastric G cells, hence increased parietal cell acid production.

The endocrine system — Answers

5   **A** = False   **B** = True   **C** = True   **D** = False   **E** = True

Endocrine cells have common cytological and behavioural characteristics and probably arise from embryonic ectoderm. Some gathered as specific organs normally secrete hormones, others are as specialized neurological tissues, e.g. adrenal medulla and hypothalamus. Tumours of these secrete excess target hormone, independent of trophic factors and feedback onto the normal endocrine axis to suppress normal endocrine tissue. However, some cells scattered through tissue of non-ectodermal origin, e.g. pancreas, gut, whether or not they normally secrete hormones in measured amounts, may do so in excess if they have become neoplastic, e.g. glucagonomas, gastrinomas, carcinoid. Finally, some scattered cells apparently non-secretory normally and not originating from endocrine tissue, may secrete hormones foreign to the host tissue, inappropriately.

6   **A** = True   **B** = True   **C** = True   **D** = True   **E** = True

All the above neoplasms take up amines and secrete hormonally active peptides, whether they do so or not normally. Hence the tissues partake in the diffuse endocrine (APUD) system. Neuroendocrine parafollicular thyroid tissue secretes calcitonin. APUD cells in adrenal medulla secrete the catecholamines, adrenaline and noradrenaline. Phaeochromocytoma, most common in fourth and fifth decades, and neuroblastomas most common in childhood, produce excess of these and may arise from medullary or extramedullary tissues. Gastrin, normally secreted by gastric antral G cells, may be produced in excess by G cell tumours of the pancreas. Ectopic hormone production (always inappropriate whereas the converse is not true) most commonly arises from small cell carcinoma of bronchus elaborating a variety of hormone types.

8 HAEMATOLOGY

1 The following cells are of the myeloid cell line
   A T lymphocytes
   B Platelets
   C Promonocyte
   D Basophilic normoblast
   E Burr cells (acanthocytes)

2 The normal red cell
   A Is biconvex
   B Has only haemoglobin within the cell membrane
   C Has a normal mean corpuscular volume (MCV) of 80–100 fl
   D Has a normal mean corpuscular haemoglobin content of 15–20 pg
   E Is an erythroblast

3 The following are recognized associations with anaemias
   A Megaloblastic anaemia and chronic atrophic gastritis
   B Hypochromic microcytic anaemia and the post-operative period
   C Pernicious anaemia and fatty change in the kidneys
   D Iron deficiency anaemia and gastrectomy
   E *Diphyllobothrium latum* and megaloblastic anaemia

4 In individuals with sickle cell disease
   A Splenomegaly is common
   B Gall stones are common
   C Red cell survival is prolonged
   D Osteomyelitis is most commonly caused by *Salmonella*
   E Sickling may be precipitated by fluid overload

5 The following may cause haemolysis
   A α-Methyl-dopa
   B Glucose-6-phosphate oxidase deficiency
   C Splenectomy
   D A Rhesus positive foetus with a Rhesus negative mother
   E Blackwater fever

6 The following may cause polycythaemia
   A Myelofibrosis
   B Trisomy 21 (Down's syndrome)
   C Hepatocellular carcinoma
   D Thrombocytosis
   E Myelodysplasia

7 Thrombocytopaenia
   A Will normally cause ecchymoses
   B Will normally cause petechiae
   C Will normally predispose to haemarthrosis
   D Becomes symptomatic at a platelet count of <50,000/mm^3 (5×10^9/litres)
   E May occur following aspirin ingestion

HAEMATOLOGY – Questions

8   The following may cause thrombocytopaenia
    A   Blood transfusion
    B   High altitude
    C   Vitamin B_{12} deficiency
    D   Henoch–Schonlein disease
    E   HIV infection

9   The following cause thrombocytosis
    A   Adrenaline
    B   Splenectomy
    C   Trauma
    D   Pregnancy
    E   Hyperlipidaemia

10 Platelets
    A   Have a normal life-span of approximately 20 days
    B   Survive for about one week in stored blood for transfusion
    C   Release serotonin on contact with collagen
    D   Undergo diapedesis when activated
    E   Contain ADP

11 Regarding the clotting system
    A   Factor XII is part of the intrinsic system
    B   Factor III is part of the intrinsic system
    C   Cleavage of fibrinogen to fibrin activates platelets
    D   Factor VII is common to both pathways
    E   Calcium is required for clotting to occur

12 The following predispose to thrombosis
    A   Tay–Sachs disease
    B   Parturition
    C   Protein C deficiency
    D   Stasis
    E   Pancreatic carcinoma

13 The following are found in hyperacute transplant rejection
    A   It may begin up to one week following transplantation
    B   A grossly cyanotic organ
    C   A mononuclear interstitial infiltrate
    D   Arteriolar intimal fibrosis
    E   Parenchymal infarction

14 Anaphylaxis
    A   Is an example of a type II hypersensitivity reaction
    B   May produce hives
    C   May lead to bronchial asthma
    D   Is mediated by IgA antibodies
    E   Occurs following initial exposure to antigen

HAEMATOLOGY – Questions

15 The following cells express MHC II (MHC = major histocompatibility complex) antigens
   A B lymphocytes
   B Reticulocytes
   C Activated T lymphocytes
   D Fibroblasts
   E Renal tubular epithelium

16 The following lead to impairment of neutrophil function
   A Sickle cell disease
   B Diabetes mellitus
   C Osteopetrosis
   D Corticosteroids
   E Bernard–Soulier syndrome

17 Transfusion
   A Anti-leucocyte antibodies rarely cause serious effects
   B Type O Rhesus negative is the universal recipient
   C IgG is the predominant anti-A and anti-B immunoglobulin
   D Pyrexia during blood transfusion indicates that transfusion should be slowed down
   E Current recommendations for transfusion are a haemoglobin of <10 g/dl

18 Hodgkin's lymphoma
   A Commonly involves Waldeyer's ring (pharyngeal lymph nodes)
   B Diagnosis requires positive identification of Reed–Sternberg cells
   C Has a female preponderance
   D Often presents as a maxillary mass
   E Generalized lymphadenopathy is common

19 An INR (international normalized ratio) requires the following substrates
   A Citrated blood
   B Platelet phospholipid
   C A glass tube
   D Tissue thromboplastin
   E Temperature of 36°C

20 Activated partial thromboplastin time (APTT or KCCT) is prolonged in
   A Alcoholic liver disease
   B Heparin therapy
   C Christmas disease (factor IX deficiency)
   D Warfarin therapy
   E Paracetamol toxicity

21 In haemophilia
    A   Inheritance is sex-linked
    B   Only women can be carriers
    C   Factor VIII is not produced
    D   Introduces resistance to malaria
    E   Haemarthrosis is common

HAEMATOLOGY — Answers 45

1 **A** = False **B** = True **C** = True **D** = False **E** = False

Lymphoid precursors produce lymphocytes only. As a general rule all other blood cells are myeloid. The normoblast is a red cell precursor. A burr cell is a type of damaged red blood cell.

2 **A** = False **B** = False **C** = True **D** = False **E** = False

The normal red cell is biconcave with a volume of 80–100 fl and a haemoglobin content of 27–34 pg. As well as containing haemoglobin the red cell also possesses an actin cytoskeleton abnormalities of which can lead to conditions like hereditary elliptocytosis and spherocytosis. All nucleated red blood cells are grouped as erythroblasts as the normal mature erythrocyte does not fall into this category; E is false.

3 **A** = True **B** = False **C** = True **D** = True **E** = True

The stomach is required to produce HCl and intrinsic factor from parietal cells. These are essential to the absorption of iron and vitamin B_{12}, respectively. Atrophic gastritis particularly causes B_{12} deficiency and therefore megaloblastic anaemia. Post-operative anaemia is due to blood loss causing red cell morphology to initially be normal and then macrocytic during the ensuing reticulocytosis. Pernicious anaemia is classically associated with visceral fatty degeneration. Gastrectomy leads to loss of HCl production and intestinal hurry through the duodenum where most of the iron is absorbed in the ferrous state. *Diphyllobothrium latum* is a fish tapeworm which causes B_{12} deficiency and hence megaloblastic anaemia, for unknown reasons in Finland only.

4 **A** = False **B** = True **C** = False **D** = True **E** = False

Sickle cell disease is due to homozygogeneity for a point cell mutation on the β-globin chain. This results in the production of the abnormal haemoglobin HbS and not the normal HbA. Reduced HbS is insoluble and precipitates in the red blood cell resulting in abnormal cell morphlogy. Sickling crises may be precipitated by dehydration and hypoxia. Aplastic crises may also occur and in children often follow parvovirus infection. Autoinfarction of the spleen almost invariably occurs by adulthood, and individuals with sickle cell disease are predisposed to sepsis particularly pneumococcal meningitis and *Salmonella* osteomyelitis. Chronic haemolysis leads to pigment-type gall stones as red cell survival is reduced from 100 to 20 days.

5 **A** = True **B** = False **C** = False **D** = True **E** = True

α-Methyl-dopa is associated with warm IgG autoantibodies and haemolysis. It is glucose-6-phosphate dehydrogenase deficiency which causes haemolysis with exposure to antimalarials and other oxidants. Splenectomy reduces sequestration of abnormal cells and is particularly therapeutic in hereditary spherocytosis. If a Rhesus negative mother has a Rhesus positive foetus then haemolysis may occur in the foetus, particularly in the event of previous maternal exposure to the rhesus antigen. Blackwater fever occurs in chronic malaria with variable quinine compliance and is the result of massive haemolysis.

46 HAEMATOLOGY – Answers

6   **A** = False   **B** = True   **C** = True   **D** = False   **E** = True

Polycythaemia is defined as an increase in red cell concentration. It may be relative or absolute. In stress and dehydration polycythaemia is relative. Absolute polycythaemia may be primary or secondary. The primary type is due to a myeloid stem cell abnormality causing polycythaemia rubra vera or a myeloproliferative disorder. The secondary may be physiological in response to: lung disease, high altitude or cyanotic heart disease (as often is the case in trisomy 21) or non-physiological secondary to erythropoietin secreting tumours such as renal cell carcinoma and hepatocellular carcinoma.

7   **A** = False   **B** = True   **C** = False   **D** = False   **E** = False

Thrombocytopaenia generally becomes symptomatic at platelet counts of <20,000/mm^3 (<20 × 10^9/litres) these may include petechiae and prolonged bleeding time. Ecchymoses may occur but are more commonly found in association with clotting factor pathologies as is the case with haemarthrosis. Aspirin reduces thromboxane production and therefore platelet aggregation but has no direct effect on platelet numbers.

8   **A** = True   **B** = False   **C** = True   **D** = False   **E** = True

Thrombocytopaenia may be due to decreased platelet production, decreased platelet survival or dilutional factors. There are no functioning platelets in transfused blood which has been stored for more than 24 h, therefore large volume transfusions may dilute existing platelets. Platelet production is decreased in aplastic anaemia, leukaemias, myelofibrosis, vitamin B$_{12}$ and folate deficiency. Platelet survival is reduced by sequestration in the spleen, autoantibody production, HIV infection and microangiopathic haemolytic anaemia. Henoch–Schonlein pupura is caused by the widespread deposition of immune complexes causing abdominal pain, arthralgia, glomerulonephritis and a purpuric rash. The platelet count is usually normal.

9   **A** = True   **B** = True   **C** = True   **D** = False   **E** = False

Adrenaline causes a 50% increase in platelet count in non-splenectomized individuals. The absence of response in splenectomized patients suggests splenic storage of platelets. Splenectomy prevents removal of effete platelets and increases the circulating count. Response to trauma includes rises in white cell count and platelet count (this may be adrenaline mediated). Although the white cell count rises moderately in pregnancy the platelet count normally falls. *Post partum* the platelet count normally shows a moderate rise. Hyperlipidaemia does not increase platelet count but does increase platelet adhesiveness.

10   **A** = False   **B** = False   **C** = True   **D** = False   **E** = True

The normal life-span of a platelet is 9–12 days. In stored blood for transfusion this is shortened to 24 h. On contact with collagen, endotoxin and antibody–antigen complexes platelets secrete ADP and serotonin, they put out pseudopodia and aggregate. Platelet factor, a membrane phospholipid, is unmasked to produce binding sites for clotting factors V and VIII. Diapedesis is a characteristic of migrating leucocytes.

HAEMATOLOGY – Answers

11 A = True B = False C = False D = False E = True

The clotting sequence is a cascade in which inactive zymogens are activated sequentially into proteolytic enzymes which selectively activate the next zymogen in the cascade. The intrinsic pathway begins with activation of factor XII and the extrinsic pathway is triggered by tissue thromboplastin release into the blood (factor III). Factor X is common to both pathways factor VII being part of the extrinsic pathway. Conversion of prothrombin (factor II) to thrombin activates platelets. Calcium (factor IV) and phospholipids act as co-enzymes in the clotting cascade.

12 A = False B = True C = True D = True E = True

Tay–Sachs disease is an hereditary mucopolysaccharidosis and has no effect on thrombogenicity. The second most common cause of *post partum* maternal mortality is pulmonary embolus. Protein C is a natural anticoagulant similar in function to anti-thrombin III. Stasis is one factor involved in Virchow's triad. For unknown reasons pancreatic carcinoma and several other malignancies are associated with thrombophlebitis migrans.

13 A = False B = True C = False D = False E = True

Hyperacute rejection occurs from within minutes to up to 48 h after transplantation. Pre-existing circulating antibodies induce complement and antibody-dependent cell mediated cytotoxicity (ADCC). The net result of this is arteriolar fibrinoid necrosis, parenchymal infarction and a cyanotic organ. Mononuclear cells and intimal fibrosis are characteristically seen in chronic rejection.

14 A = False B = True C = True D = False E = False

Anaphylaxis is a rapidly developing immunological reaction occurring after a combination of antigen with IgE antibody bound to mast cells or basophils in a previously sensitized individual. It may occur as a local phenomenon as seen with hives, hayfever and bronchial asthma or may have systemic effects leading rapidly to anaphylactic shock.

15 A = True B = False C = True D = False E = False

All cells express MHC I antigens. Antigen presenting cells express MHC II. These include Langerhans cells in the skin, macrophages B lymphocytes and activated T lymphocytes.

16 A = False B = True C = False D = True E = False

Sickle cell disease impairs complement activity. Osteopetrosis causes a reduction in bone marrow and therefore reduces neutrophil numbers but not function. Bernard–Soulier syndrome affects platelet aggregation.

17 A = True B = False C = False D = False E = False

O negative carries no A, B or Rhesus antigen and is therefore a universal donor. IgM is the predominant anti-A anti-B immunoglobulin. Anti-leucocyte antibodies rarely cause more than fever, however initially this is clinically indistinguishable from a major transfusion reaction, and current recommendations are to cease such transfusion. Current indications for transfusion are symptomatic anaemia or a haemoglobin of <8 g/dl, these vary considerably between units.

HAEMATOLOGY – Answers

18 A = False B = True C = False D = False E = False

Diagnosis of Hodgkin's lymphoma requires the presence of the Reed–Sternberg cell on histological examination plus other features. Reed–Sternberg cells *per se* are not pathognomonic of Hodgkin's lymphoma and are also seen in infectious mononucleosis and non-Hodgkin's lymphoma. Hodgkin's lymphoma has no clear male:female preponderance although the nodular sclerosing variant classically affects young women. Involvement of Waldeyer's ring and generalized lymphadenopathy are more usually seen in non-Hodgkin's lymphoma. A maxillary mass is classically seen in Burkitt's lymphoma.

19 A = True B = False C = False D = True E = True

For prothrombin time measurement test plasma, tissue thromboplastin and calcium solution are incubated at 37°C. This is compared to a control and a ratio (INR) can be calculated. A glass tube and platelet phospholipid are used to estimate the partial thromboplastin time, reflecting the requirements of the intrinsic system for surface contact and platelets.

20 A = True B = True C = True D = True E = True

The APTT is a measure of the activity of the intrinsic and common pathways. That is, every clotting factor except factor VII. The liver produces every clotting factor except Von Willebrand factor. Compromise will therefore affect both limbs of the clotting cascade. Warfarin affects manufacture of clotting factors II, VII, IX and X. Christmas disease involves factor IX.

21 A = True B = False C = False D = False E = True

Haemophilia is a sex-linked recessive disease. Haemarthrosis is a common problem; a daughter of a carrier woman and an affected man will be affected. Factor VIII is produced but is ineffective. Sickle cell disease but not haemophilia aids in resistance to malaria.

9 CNS PATHOLOGY

1. Intracranial calcification is associated with
   - A Craniopharyngioma
   - B Intracerebral haemorrhage
   - C Meningioma
   - D Oligodendroglioma
   - E Staphylococcal abscess

2. The following produce well circumscribed lesions
   - A Astrocytoma
   - B Oligodendroglioma
   - C Ependymoma
   - D Metastatic tumours
   - E Intracerebral haemorrhages

3. Processes following peripheral nerve section may include
   - A Chromatolysis
   - B Segmental demyelination
   - C Wallerian degeneration
   - D Traumatic neuroma
   - E Axonal regeneration of 1 mm per day

4. Regarding the diagnosis of brain stem death
   - A Brain stem encephalitis may cause death
   - B Apnoea breathing oxygen is required
   - C Decerebrate posture is suggestive of brain stem death
   - D The oculocephallic reflex must be tested
   - E Mydriasis is required

5. With regard to anaesthetic agents
   - A The minimum alveolar concentration (MAC) of an inhalational anaesthetic agent is inversely proportional to its lipid solubility
   - B Thiopentone causes hypotension and a reduced cardiac output
   - C Ketamine usage as an IV induction agent can produce hypertension and tachycardia
   - D Suxamethonium commonly causes muscular fasciculation
   - E Atropine acts well as an antisialogogue when given as a premedicant

6. Regarding anaesthetic/analgesics
   - A Patients with an epidural catheter *in situ* are best nursed supine
   - B The maximum safe dosage of 2% plain lignocaine in a 90 kg man is 13.5 ml
   - C Bupivacaine is the agent of choice in Bier's block
   - D Activity of local anaesthetics may be reduced in the presence of local infection
   - E Abducent nerve palsy may be a complication of spinal anaesthesia

CNS PATHOLOGY – Questions

1 A = True B = False C = True D = True E = False

Craniopharyngiomas are tumours of remnants of Rathke's pouch, part solid and part cystic, 75% of which calcify in the vicinity of stella turcica. Oligodendrogliomas are both haemorrhagic and calcific, mostly microscopically but occasionally sequestrating huge amounts of the latter. Arising from the meninges and indenting the brain, meningiomas are often gritty in texture because of the psammoma bodies they contain. Haemorrhage into the brain is followed by influx of macrophages and phagocytosis of blood pigments resulting in haemosiderin-laden cells once resorption of extravasated blood has occurred leaving a slit-like cavity. Although calcification is a common intracranial reaction to injury, in the brain the normal niduses for calcification do not occur.

2 A = False B = True C = True D = True E = True

Astrocytes are stellate cells with plentiful fibrillary processes forming a cellular framework upon which neuronal and neuroglial structures lie. Hence these tumours are typically ill-defined and infiltrative. Oligodendrocytes secrete myelin. Ependymal cells line ventricles and partake in choroid plexus formation. Although these tumours are solid and well circumscribed, they often lie on the floor of the fourth ventricle adjacent to the brain stem structures and their extirpation is a problem. The sharp demarcation of metastatic tumours may be of diagnostic value in separating them from intracranial primaries on scanning radiography, usually lying in the junction between grey and white matter with surrounding oedema. Haemorrhage most often occurs along planes of cleavage.

3 A = True B = False C = True D = True E = True

With nerve transection, the distal axon and myelin sheath disintegrate, digested by Schwann cells. Proximal degeneration of both axon and sheath occurs to the previous node of Ranvier. This is Wallerian degeneration, not segmental demyelination which is the loss of individual isolated myelin internodes with axonal preservation. Axonal cell body reaction may occur in response, with paling of the cytoplasm (chromatolysis) and swelling. Regeneration occurs with axonal sprouting from the cut ends, the direction of which is governed by the perineural sheaths if they have not been disrupted. Some regeneration of function may ensue should they reach their target end organ, otherwise the tangled axons produce at hyperaesthetic painful area.

4 A = False B = False C = False D = False E = False

In the presence of irremedial structural brain damage and apnoeic coma, and in the absence of drug, metabolic, physical or endocrine abnormalities, testing of brain stem reflexes may be considered. The standard tests are the corneal reflex (absent to a strong stimulus), pupillary response (absent to a bright light), caloric stimulation (no eye movements with injection of iced water into the auditory meatus), painful stimuli to the trigeminal area (no response), gag reflex (no gag or cough). Apnoea on oxygen is insufficient; it must be with a pCO_2 of at least 6.65 kPa for 10 min. Current guidelines state that testing should be carried out by one consultant and one senior registrar and repeated after a length of time between 30 min and 24 h.

CNS PATHOLOGY – Questions

5 **A** = False   **B** = True   **C** = True   **D** = True   **E** = True

The MAC is directly proportional to the lipid solubility of on inhalational anaesthetic agent. It is the alveolar concentration at which 50% of patients do not move in response to a surgical stimulus. Thiopentone is the most popularly used IV induction agent and causes peripheral vasodilatation and venous pooling, hence hypotension and a reduced cardiac output. Ketamine can cause hypertension and tachycardia, is an effective analgesic and does not cause respiratory depression. Suxamethonium does cause fasciculation as it is a partial agonist for ACh at the neuromuscular junction. Two major problems associated with suxamethonium are suxamethonium apnoea and malignant hyperpyrexia. Predisposition to both are inherited as autosomal recessive and dominant traits respectively. Atropine has two main uses: firstly it reduces secretions and secondly works well as an anti-vagal drug protecting the heart from reflex bradycardia induced by anti-cholinesterases given for reversal of muscle relaxation.

6 **A** = False   **B** = True   **C** = False   **D** = True   **E** = True

Patients with an epidural catheter *in situ* may suffer respiratory depression if they are not nursed upright. This tends to follow 6–8 hours after lying the patient flat due to accumulation of the agent used. The maximum safe dose of lignocaine is 3 mg/kg, therefore 13.5 ml of a 2% plain solution in a 90 kg man is the maximum safe dosage. Prilocaine 0.5% plain is the agent of choice for Bier's block as it is the least cardiotoxic agent and the safest should the cuff deflate. Activity of local anaesthetics is reduced in the presence of local infection due to a reduction in local pH causing reduced anaesthetic dissociation and membrane solubility. Abducent nerve palsy may follow spinal anaesthesia due to the long intracranial part of the sixth nerve being stretched over the wing of the sphenoid when an excessive volume of CSF is lost.

10 Microbiology, Sterilization and Disinfection

1. Regarding infection with *Mycobacterium tuberculosis* (TB)
   A. There is an increased susceptibility in patients with silicosis
   B. The organism fluoresces with auramine staining in ultraviolet light
   C. The initial response to infection with *Mycobacterium tuberculosis* involves epitheloid cells
   D. Characteristic caseation necrosis is due to release of mycobacterial endotoxin
   E. Ectopic calcification of a single peripheral lung field lesion on CXR may show the presence of a healed ghon complex

2. Regarding TB infection
   A. The Assmann focus occurs mainly in childhood TB infection
   B. Progression to cavitation may lead to increased infectivity to others
   C. Direct spread of caseous material into a bronchus may lead to tuberculous lobar pneumonia
   D. In miliary TB the patient shows a strong and florid reaction to skin inoculation
   E. The degree of protection afforded by BCG inoculation with an attenuated strain of the organism is related to the degree of hypersensitivity produced

3. With regard to *Mycobacterium leprae*
   A. *Mycobacterium leprae* has a predilection for warmer tissues
   B. *Mycobacterium leprae* is aerobic and grows slowly in culture
   C. Lepromatous leprosy has an incubation period of three to six years
   D. Lesions of lepromatous leprosy contain predominantly acid fast bacilli, foamy macrophages with lymphocytes and mast cells
   E. Erythema nodosum leprosum occurs only in the tuberculoid form of the disease

4. With respect to sarcoidosis
   A. Epitheloid granuloma formation with no central necrosis are seen
   B. Asteroid bodies are found in the cytoplasm of multinucleate giant cells in sarcoid granulomas
   C. The ocular triad of sarcoid manifestations is known as Sjogren's syndrome
   D. Hypocalcaemia may accompany sarcoidosis
   E. In the Kveim test sarcoid tissue injected intradermally produces a rapid inflammatory reaction composed of the histologically identifiable intradermal sarcoid lesions

5. In syphilitic infection
   A. *Treponema pallidum* is resistant to heat and drying
   B. In the Wasserman reaction the Wasserman antibody is an IgG molecule which reacts with lipid cell membranes
   C. In 90% of patients with primary syphilis if the disease is left untreated there is no progression to the secondary stage
   D. Condylomata lata are seen in secondary syphilis
   E. A syphilitic gumma exhibits coagulative necrosis

54 MICROBIOLOGY – Questions

6 A false positive Wassermann reaction can be found in patients with
   A Malaria
   B Tuberculosis
   C Mycoplasmal pneumonia
   D Infectious mononucleosis
   E Sarcoidosis

7 Regarding tertiary syphilis
   A Most gummatous lesions heal without scarring
   B Peri-intimal cuffing is seen in syphilitic lesions
   C Aortic regurgitation is sometimes seen in this disease
   D Hydrocephalus may be a feature
   E In tabes dorsalis organisms are readily identified in the lesions found

8 Regarding viruses
   A All DNA viruses have an eicosahedral capsid except pox viruses
   B Most DNA viruses have no envelope except herpes viruses
   C Viruses may undergo binary fission
   D The influenza virus carries a specific protein receptor for
       N-acetylneuraminic acid (NANA)
   E Viropexis is inevitable and rapid following attachment

9 Regarding viral replication
   A In DNA virus replication early proteins form structural components
   B RNA virus replication usually occurs in the host cell nucleus
   C The possession of DNA dependent, RNA polymerase is a unique property
       of retroviruses
   D During the eclipse phase of viral replication, viral particles are not detected
       in the host cell
   E Togaviruses characteristically replicate in the vascular endothelium

10 Regarding RNA viruses
    A Polio virus is an example of a picorna virus
    B Orthomyxoviruses have dsRNA
    C Minor changes in the haemoglutinins of a particular type of influenza virus
        cause antigenic shift
    D Mumps virus is similar to influenza virus in that it also has haemagglutinins
        and neuraminidase on its capsid
    E Burkitt's lymphoma has been associated with an RNA virus

11 With regard to hepatitis
    A Hepatitis A virus is a DNA-containing virus
    B Hepatitis B is usually transmitted by the faecal–oral root
    C Damage to liver cells in hepatitis B infection is due to cell mediated
        immune mechanisms
    D Chronic active hepatitis is found in 50% of patients with symptomatic
        chronic hepatitis infection
    E Patients who contract hepatitis B and only suffer a subclinical infection
        causing them to have a carrier status are at no increased risk of hepatoma

MICROBIOLOGY – Questions 55

12 Viruses and neoplasia
   A The organism responsible for condylomata lata has been implicated in the aetiology of cervical cancer
   B Burkitt's lymphoma incidence is declining in those area where malaria has been eradicated
   C People expressing the sickle cell trait have an increased likelihood of developing Burkitt's lymphoma
   D Nasopharyngeal carcinoma is associated with cytomegalovirus infection
   E Protooncogenes are found in oncogenic viruses

13 *Actinomycetes israelii* infection
   A Is caused by a Gram negative bacterium
   B Is an obligate aerobe
   C Is not diagnosed by antibody demonstration
   D Is an oral commensal
   E Causes anchovy-sauce cyst formation in the liver

14 Toxoplasmosis
   A *Toxoplasma gondii* is an obligatory intracellular parasite
   B Has a positive Paul–Bunnell reaction
   C Transplacental transmission occurs during the second trimester of pregnancy
   D The cerebral spread of the disease particularly affects the walls of the lateral ventricles
   E Infection is treated with metronidazole

15 Regarding bacteria
   A Bacteria have their own mitochondria
   B Bacterial DNA is in the form of a double helical circle
   C Bacteria have a diploid genome
   D Plasmids may only replicate within bacterial cells
   E Transduction involves the uptake by bacteria of naked DNA derived from another bacterial cell

16 Regarding the diagnosis of bacterial infection
   A *Pneumococcus* has a characteristic capsule
   B *Spirochaetes* have flagellae
   C Bacterial L-forms are exquisitely sensitive to antibiotic therapy
   D *Spirochaetes* are only usually visible on dark-ground illumination
   E *Actinomycetes* consist of simple branching filaments on microscopy

17 Regarding bacteria and viruses
   A Obligate anaerobes are rich in the enzyme catalase
   B The log phase of bacterial replication precedes the lag phase
   C An anticoagulant should be added to all cytology specimens
   D Chocolate agar is particularly useful in the culture of *Haemophilus influenza*
   E CSF protein content is raised in viral meningitis

MICROBIOLOGY – Questions

18 Aseptic meningitis can commonly be caused by the following organisms
  A Poliovirus
  B Togaviruses
  C Hepatitis B virus
  D As a complication of zoster
  E *Mycobacterium tuberculosis*

19 Regarding therapy for viral disease
  A Amantadine acts by interfering with viral nucleic acid replication
  B Adenine arabinoside (ara-A, vidarabine) is the drug of choice for herpes simplex virus encephalitis
  C Acyclovir is inactive until activated by viral thymidine kinase
  D Rifampicin is used in the treatment of vaccinia infection
  E Ethambutol is used against herpes simplex virus infections

20 Regarding theatre design and procedure
  A Air filters should have pores of a diameter less than 50 μm
  B Air extractors should be at ceiling level
  C Skin shaving one day pre-operatively increases the risk of wound sepsis
  D Staphylococcal flora may be significantly reduced by routinely disinfecting the skin several days pre-operatively with hexachlorophane soaps
  E *Pseudomonas aeruginosa* is a typical contaminant of operating theatre humidifiers

21 Regarding disinfection and sterilization
  A During sterilization only vegetative forms of organisms are destroyed
  B Surgical skin preparation with iodine is an example of sterilization
  C Dry heat at 160°C for one hour provides an adequate atmosphere for sterilization
  D Tyndallization is an adequate sterilizing practice for drugs, suture material and instruments
  E Moist heat works via destructive oxidation of cell constituents

22 With regard to sterilization and disinfection
  A Theatre packs are best removed from the autoclave when still moist
  B Autoclaving may be used to sterilize parenteral crystalloid solutions
  C The Bowie–Dick test involves the disappearance of bars along the length of autoclave tape showing adequate sterilization to have occurred
  D Iodine is active both against vegatative forms of microorganisms and spores
  E Hypochlorite solutions are ineffective against viruses

23 Regarding sterilization and disinfection
  A Isopropyl alcohol is effective against both vegetative organisms and spores
  B Aldehydes (e.g. formalin/formaldehyde) are ineffective against spores
  C Chlorhexidine is effective against spores
  D Sterilization using ethylene oxide is made more rapid by adding a 10% mixture of CO_2
  E Rubber catheters may be adequately cleaned by boiling at 100°C

MICROBIOLOGY – Answers

1   **A** = True   **B** = True   **C** = False   **D** = False   **E** = False

There is indeed an increased susceptibility to become infected with *Mycobacterium tuberculosis* in patients with silicosis, diabetes, the immunocompromised, debilitated or people from the Asian subcontinent. The organism fluoresces with auramine staining and ultraviolet light. Other methods of identification include acid fastness and Ziehl–Neelsen staining. The initial response to infection with *Mycobacterium tuberculosis* is acute inflammation involving PMNLs and macrophages which present mycobacterial antigens to T helper cells. Epithelioid cell transformation occurs later. Caseating necrosis is due to release of lysosomal enzymes from macrophages. Calcification of a single peripheral lung field lesion on chest X-ray in a patient previously infected with tuberculosis is dystrophic rather than ectopic in nature. This is a ghon focus, a ghon complex is the parenchymal lesion and the local lymph node infection.

2   **A** = False   **B** = True   **C** = False   **D** = False   **E** = False

The Assmann focus is seen mainly in adult TB where there is little lymphatic involvement. This is found in the subapical region of the upper lobe of the lung. Erosion of the caseous material into a bronchus may cause an increase in oxygen tension, bacterial multiplication and infectivity to others. Erosion into bronchial vessels may cause massive haemoptysis and hypovolaemic shock. Direct spread of caseous material into a bronchus may lead to tuberculosis bronchopneumonia. In miliary TB no skin reaction is seen. These patients have diminished hypersensitivity. The degree of protection afforded by BCG inoculation is not proportionate to the degree of hypersensitivity produced.

3   **A** = False   **B** = False   **C** = False   **D** = True   **E** = False

Mycobacterium leprae prefers cooler tissues such as skin, nasal mucosa, peripheral nerves and testis. It is an obligatory intracellular parasite unlike *Mycobacterium tuberculosis* which is aerobic and grows slowly in culture. Tuberculoid leprosy has an incubation period of 3–6 years. For lepromatous leprosy this is 10–20 years. Erythema nodosum leprosum is found in lepromatous leprosy and is due to immune complex deposition in subcutaneous blood vessels causing tender subcutaneous nodules.

4   **A** = True   **B** = True   **C** = False   **D** = False   **E** = False

Sarcoid is most common in Sweden and may affect any tissue, particularly the lungs, liver and spleen. Bony involvement may lead to osteitis cystica multiplex. Calcified asteroid bodies are seen but are not diagnostic of sarcoid. The uveal tract, lacrimal gland and salivary gland triad seen in sarcoid is known as Heerfordt's syndrome. Hypercalcaemia may accompany sarcoidosis due to an increased sensitivity to vitamin D. The Kveim test produces an extremely slow reaction.

5   **A** = False   **B** = False   **C** = False   **D** = True   **E** = True

Treponema pallidum is very sensitive to drying. The Wassermann antibody is an IgM. In 50% of untreated case of primary syphilis there is no progression to the secondary stage of the disease. Condylomata lata are seen in secondary syphilis and affect the mucocutaneous areas of the anus, vulva and perineum. Snail track ulcers are seen in the mouth and pharynx. Cell outlines in the centre of a gumma are still maintained unlike caseating tuberculous lesions.

MICROBIOLOGY – Answers

6 A = True   B = False   C = True   D = True   E = False

False positive Wassermann reactions are commonly found with malaria, glandular fever, leprosy, trypanosomiasis, mycoplasmal pneumonia, certain auto-immune haemolytic anaemias, SLE, other treponemal disorders, e.g. yaws, pinta and bejel and some coxsackie-B virus infections.

7 A = False   B = False   C = True   D = True   E = False

All gummatous lesions heal with coarse scarring and fibrosis especially lesions affecting the liver, testis, skin and bone. Periadventitial cuffing occurs in small blood vessels in syphilitic lesions due to accumulation of fibroblasts, macrophages and lymphocytes. This causes stenosis of small vessels. Aortic regurgitation is seen due to small vessel disease of the vasa vasorum of the root of the aorta and this can lead to aneurysm formation in the ascending aorta. Cranial involvement by gummatous lesions may obstruct the foramina of the fourth ventricle blocking CSF outflow and leading to hydrocephalus. Cerebral manifestations of syphilitic infection include chronic meningitis and parenchymatous neurosyphilis. The latter comprises two distinct syndromes; tabes dorsalis and general paresis of the insane. In GPI treponemes are easily isolated. However, this is not true in tabes dorsalis.

8 A = True   B = True   C = False   D = False   E = False

Most RNA viruses have a helical capsid. DNA viruses have an eicosahaedral capsid except pox viruses. Most DNA viruses have no envelope except herpes virus. Most RNA viruses are enveloped except picorna and reoviruses. Viruses, unlike bacteria do not undergo binary fision. Host cells have the N-acetylneuraminic acid receptor, the influenza virus attaches to them via a haemagglutinin binding site carried on its envelope. Viropexis is temperature and energy dependent and is inhibited by metabolic poisons. It is not an inevitable consequence of attachment.

9 A = False   B = False   C = False   D = True   E = True

Early proteins in DNA virus replication are DNA synthesis proteins. Late proteins constitute the material from which capsomeres are made. With the exception of orthomyxoviruses (e.g. influenza), RNA virus replication occurs within the host cell cytoplasm unlike DNA virus replication which occurs within the nucleus. The unique property of retroviruses is the possession of reverse transcriptase or RNA-dependent DNA polymerase. The eclipse phase of viral replication varies from virus to virus and precedes viral release by budding or lysis. Togaviruses cause yellow fever, haemorrhagic fevers and encephalitides.

10 A = True   B = False   C = False   D = True   E = False

The picorna group of viruses comprise entero and rhino viruses. Enteroviruses include polio virus, coxsackie virus and echo virus. Rhinoviruses cause the common cold. Orthomyxoviruses have single stranded RNA and cause influenza. Minor changes in the haemoglutinins of influenza virus cause antigenic drift. Antigenic shift is due to a more fundamental reorganization of the antigenic make up of the viral strain. Mumps, measles and croup are paramyxoviruses. Influenza is an orthomyxovirus. Burkitt's lymphoma has been associated with Epstein–Barr virus, one of the herpes group of DNA viruses.

MICROBIOLOGY – Answers

11 A = False   B = False   C = True   D = True   E = False

Hepatitis A is an RNA virus. Hepatitis B contains small dsDNA. Hepatitis A is transmitted by the faecal–oral root. Hepatitis B is usually transmitted by i.v. innoculation, tatooing and anal or vaginal intercourse. Hepatitis B virus is not directly responsible for the pathological features of the disease, these are due to the mechanisms of viral elimination. Chronic active hepatitis is found in 50% of patients with symptomatic chronic hepatitis infection. The other half have chronic persistent hepatitis, this is the persistence of virus in liver cells with no evidence of continuing liver damage. There is an increased risk associated both with chronic hepatitis and the carrier state.

12 A = False   B = True   C = False   D = False   E = False

Treponema pallidum causes condylomata lata as a manifestation of secondary syphilis and is not associated with cervical cancer. Condylomata accuminata or genital warts are caused by the papilloma viruses, members of the papova virus group all of which have been associated with malignancy. Epstein–Barr virus causes Burkitt's lymphoma which is strikingly circumscribed to areas where malaria is endemic. The sickle cell trait is protective against malaria and also Epstein–Barr virus-induced Burkitt's lymphoma. As a tendency towards developing Burkitt's is brought about by a malaria-induced failure of immune surveillance. Nasopharyngeal carcinoma is associated with Epstein–Barr virus and the genetic susceptibility (HLA-A2 MHC). These two factors explain why South China's Kwantung province has the highest incidence of this disease. Protooncogenes are normal cellular viral oncogene precursors.

13 A = False   B = False   C = True   D = True   E = False

Sixty-five percent of actinomycosis is cervico-facial, 20% ileo-caecal and the remainder is pulmonary. The characteristic appearance is of multiple pin head, yellow/grey abscesses in the neck. Treatment is with penicillin. Prognosis is good in the cervical type but poor in the pulmonary and abdominal variants of the disease. It is caused by a Gram positive anaerobic or at most microaerophilic bacterium. It can be identified by anaerobic culture on blood agar then crushed between two slides and stained. Branching filaments are characteristically seen. It is a normal oral commensal, especially in carious teeth. Actinomycosis causes honeycomb liver. Anchovy-sauce cysts are seen in amoebic infection.

14 A = True   B = False   C = False   D = True   E = False

Cats are the definitive host of the organism which is an obligatory intracellular parasite. The disease shows prominent lymphadenopathy similar to infectious mononucleosis. However, the Paul–Bunnell test is negative. Transplacental transmission usually occurs during the first trimester of pregnancy. Cerebral spread of the disease characteristically affects the walls of the lateral ventricles which leads to necrosis and calcification later in life. Sulphonamides or pyrimethamine (especially sulphadizine) are the treatment of choice for toxoplasmal infection.

MICROBIOLOGY – Answers

15 **A** = False **B** = True **C** = False **D** = False **E** = False

Bacteria have no endoplasmic reticulum and no mitochondria, all necessary enzymes are contained in their cytoplasmic membrane. Bacteria have a haploid genome, they are prokaryotes. Plasmids are small particles of circular dsDNA usually found in bacteria and can replicate either in the bacterium or on their own as separate entities outside the bacterial cell. Transformation involves the uptake by bacteria of naked DNA derived from another bacterial cell. Transduction involves the transfer of genetic material from a donor cell to a recipient cell by way of a viral vector.

16 **A** = True **B** = False **C** = False **D** = True **E** = True

Pneumococcus, *Klebsiella*, *Clostridium perfringens* and *Bacillus anthracis* all have a characteristic capsule. *Spirochaetes* are the only motile bacteria that lack flagellae. Bacterial L-forms are cell wall deficient bacterial variants and regardless of the antibiotic sensitivity of their parent organism they are penicillin resistant and hence are easily isolated in patients on penicillin or cephalosporin therapy. Some L-forms are stable, others revert to the parent form once the inducing agent is removed.

17 **A** = False **B** = False **C** = True **D** = True **E** = True

Obligate anaerobes are intolerant of oxygen since oxygen produces damaging peroxides inactivated by the enzyme catalase which these organisms lack. The order of bacterial replication is lag, logarithmic, stationary and decline. Anticoagulants should be added to all cytology specimens, for example, potassium oxalate. Chocolate agar is blood agar heated to 80°C for approximately 1 min. The haematinin (X factor) produced haemoglobin breakdown is useful in the growth of *Haemophilus influenzae*. CSF protein content is raised both in bacterial and viral meningitis.

18 **A** = True **B** = True **C** = False **D** = True **E** = False

The following agents can cause aseptic meningitis enterovirus including poliovirus, togaviruses, lymphocytic choriomeningitis virus, bunyaviruses, herpes simplex virus and occasionally zoster, vaccinia, mumps, measles, influenza and chickenpox.

19 **A** = False **B** = True **C** = True **D** = True **E** = False

Idoxuridine inhibits viral nucleic acid replication in vaccinia and herpes simplex virus infections. Ara-A, vidarabine is the treatment of choice for herpes simplex virus encephalitis infection, it acts by inhibiting DNA polymerase. Acyclovir has selective toxicity against viral infected cells as it is inactive until activated by viral thymidine kinase. Rifampicin is useful in the treatment of vaccinia by preventing the final assembly of viral particles. Ethambutol is useless against herpes simplex virus infection, its main use is as an anti-tuberculous drug.

20 **A** = False **B** = False **C** = True **D** = True **E** = True

Theatre air intakes should be at the ceiling level and should have filters with pores of 5 μm diameter as bacteria are usually attached to dust particles of a diameter greater than 5 μm. Air extractors should be at ground level. The practice of shaving skin several days pre-operatively can cause bacterial colonization of slightly damaged skin around the operative site and increase the risks of wound sepsis.

MICROBIOLOGY – Answers

Skin shaving immediately prior to surgery has no deleterious effects. Repetitive daily washing with hexachlorophane soap can be used significantly to reduce staphylococcal skin flora especially in orthopaedic practice. *Pseudomonas* is a typical humidification system contaminant.

21 A = False   B = False   C = True   D = False   E = False

During disinfection only vegetative forms of organisms are destroyed. In sterilization both vegetative forms and spores are destroyed. Surgical skin preparation with iodine is an example of disinfection. Dry heat at 160°C for 1 h does create an adequate atmosphere for sterilization, however, it damages fabrics and rubber and is therefore best used for glassware. Moist heat is much more rapidly effective. Tyndallization is the practice of steaming a solution for 20 min on three successive days in the hope that all spores will have become vegetative forms during this time. However, it is only of use in sterilizing media in which spores can germinate easily. Dry heat works via destructive oxidation of cell constituents, whereas moist heat destroys microorganisms by denaturing and coagulating cellular enzymes and proteins.

22 A = True   B = True   C = False   D = True   E = False

Moisture is easily penetrated by bacteria, therefore damp autoclaved packs should be left until thoroughly dry before removal from the autoclave. Autoclaving may be used to sterilize i.v. crystalloid solutions, also dressings, theatre clothes, rubber and metal instruments. In the Bowie–Dick test, bars appear over the length of autoclave tape showing adequate sterilization to have occurred. A solution of 2.5% iodine, 2.5% potassium iodide in 90% ethanol is the most effective manner in which iodine can be administered. Hypochlorite solutions are particularly effective against viruses, especially hepatitis B virus.

23 A = False   B = False   C = False   D = False   E = True

Isopropyl alcohol is only active against vegetative forms of organisms, whereas aldehydes are effective both against spores and vegetative forms. Glutaraldehyde, in particular, is used to sterilize instruments which cannot be autoclaved. Chlorhexidine is not effective against spores but it is particularly effective against Gram positive vegetative organisms, e.g. staphylococci. Ethylene oxide sterilization is made safer by adding a 10% mixture of CO_2 but not more rapid, increasing ambient temperature from 20–25°C up to 50–60°C reduces sterilization time from 18 to 4 h. As spore-forming organisms do not cause UTIs, boiling rubber catheters in water at 100°C is an adequate method of cleansing them.

11 ONCOLOGY

1. Chemical carcinogens may act by
   - A Inducing changes in the cells genome
   - B Initiation: the transformation of a cell into an autonomous structure
   - C Promotion: the gaining of immortality and autonomy by the cell
   - D Metabolism within the body into active molecules
   - E Releasing ionizing radiation to cell constituents during metabolism

2. Initiation and promotion of oncogenesis
   - A Chemical carcinogens are able to bind to and alter the DNA structure within the nucleus if they are promoters
   - B Initiating and promoting agents may cause their effects if applied many years apart or in any order
   - C The carcinogen acts by altering proto-oncogenes or recessive cancer genes, which are responsible for cell growth and differentiation
   - D 'Mutagenesis' is a synonym for chemical-induced initiation of oncogenesis
   - E Cellular attempts at DNA repair are generally ineffective against mutagens

3. Polycyclic aromatic hydrocarbons
   - A Do not require metabolism to induce initiation
   - B Are classed as 'ultimate carcinogens'
   - C Require the activity of microsomal enzymes for their actions in carcinogenesis
   - D Are strong electrophobic reagents exerting their effects by interacting with the cell's DNA
   - E Are poor carcinogens, in as much as, they rarely cause malignant transformation

4. The formation of bladder tumours by aromatic amine compounds
   - A Requires repeated metabolism to the compound within the body
   - B Is caused by the products of liver metabolism interacting directly with the bladder mucosa cells
   - C Is enhanced by the fact that humans lack urinary glucuronidase
   - D Produce malignant change without the action of promoting agents
   - E Is an example of enzymatic activation of a substance to a carcinogen

5. Radiation-induced carcinogenesis
   - A Ultraviolet radiation causes the formation of base-pair dimers leading to transcriptional errors
   - B Is associated with inhibition of cell mediated immunity
   - C Results from a failure to repair radiation induced DNA changes. This explains the high incidence of tumours in subjects with immunological disorders such as Wiskott–Aldrich syndrome
   - D Ionizing radiation is thought to cause carcinogenesis by the production of free radicals from oxygen and water molecules
   - E Chronic myeloid leukaemia is thought to be due to exposure to ionizing radiation

ONCOLOGY – Questions

6 Oncogenesis due to viruses
   A Human papilloma virus (HPV) is an RNA virus implicated in cervical cancer
   B HPV-16 and HPV-18 genetic material has been isolated in over 70% of cases of cervical cancer
   C All subsets of human papilloma virus have been implicated in neoplasia, either benign or malignant
   D The implication of HPV in carcinogenesis has been supported by DNA hybridization techniques only
   E The implication of HPV in carcinogenesis has been complicated by the fact that cell lines infected with the virus propagate the virus imperfectly leading to sporadic tumour formation

7 The role of Epstein–Barr virus in oncogenesis
   A Is proven by the fact that every patient with African Burkitt's lymphoma has antibodies to the Epsein–Barr virus
   B Is associated with immunosuppression in susceptible individuals
   C Is related to proliferation in the T-cell line leading to the increased possibility of neoplastic mutation
   D Is regional in nature: causing nasopharyngeal tumours in China and Burkitt's lymphoma in Africa
   E Is related to its production of translocations in several positions in the genome

8 Viral oncogenesis
   A RNA viral oncogenes can all be isolated from normal human genomes
   B DNA viral oncogenes code for normal cell constituents or enzymes
   C All oncogenic RNA viruses are retroviruses
   D Reverse transcriptase is a feature of RNA viruses associated with neoplastic transformation
   E Theory suggests that the similarity between c-onc sequences and v-onc sequences is related to contamination of viruses with normal human genes

9 Cellular proto-oncogenes
   A May be converted to cellular oncogenes by placement next to promoter genes
   B Are responsible for the production of cellular constituents or enzymes
   C The cellular proto-oncogene responsible for chronic myeloid leukaemia is the same as that for Burkitt's lymphoma
   D Contain similar genetic structures to viral oncogenes
   E May be converted into cellular oncogenes by gene amplification

10 The development of retinoblastoma
    A Requires the mutation of a locus on both chromosomes in the sporadic form
    B Requires translocation of a promoter gene into close proximity of the *Rb* gene
    C Is an example of malignant change arising from the loss of a suppressor gene
    D In the familial form requires no mutation as the defective gene is already present in each cell
    E Is transmitted as an autosomal recessive trait in the familial form

ONCOLOGY – Questions

11 The following evidence suggests that cancer is a 'genetic disease'
   A Chromosomal abnormalities, specific to a particular neoplasm, may be found in tumour cells
   B The effect of carcinogens on the cell is by mutagenesis of the DNA
   C The cell growth is continuous
   D Carcinogenesis is often a one-step process
   E Congenital immune deficiencies predispose to cancer development

12 Effects of neoplasms on the host
   A Benign neoplasms cause effects dependent solely on their site
   B Malignant neoplasms cause cachexia by using much of the body's energy to sustain its high turnover rate
   C Malignant tumours commonly synthesize hormones
   D The hormones produced by malignant tumours are often different to that produced by the surrounding cells
   E Paraneoplastic syndromes may cause the death of the patient before significant tumour mass is attained

13 Paraneoplastic syndromes: the following are correctly associated
   A Polycythaemia – renal carcinoma
   B Hypoglycaemia – intracranial carcinoma
   C Hypercalcaemia – bronchogenic carcinoma
   D Cushing's syndrome – bronchogenic carcinoma
   E Dermatomyositis – gastric carcinoma

14 The paraneoplastic syndromes of malignant disease
   A Occur in only 10% of patients with advanced malignant disease
   B May be produced by hormones synthesized by the tumour
   C Hormone production by the tumour is caused by failure to suppress certain elements of the cell's genetic composition
   D Hypercalcaemia indicates the presence of bony involvement, either primary or secondary
   E Myasthenia is due to released cancer antibodies cross-reacting with neuromuscular junctions in muscle fibres

15 Hypercalcaemia in malignant disease
   A Of the paraneoplastic syndromes is second only to Cushing's syndrome in frequency
   B May be due to osteolysis caused by either primary or secondary bony involvement
   C Peptides with parathyroid hormone activity may cause hypercalcaemia in ways similar to that of hyperparathyroidism
   D Transforming growth factor alpha (TGF-α) produces hypercalcaemia by suppression of normal osteoblastic activity, leading to an unbalanced loss of bone by the osteoclasts
   E Responds to the same treatment as Cushing's disease

Oncology – Questions

16 Cachexia in malignant disease
   A Is related to the size of the cancer
   B May be due to intercurrent or chronic infection in a debilitated patient
   C Is due to the nutritional drain of sustaining the enlarging cancer
   D May be related to alteration in appetite
   E May be related to the release of a lymphocyte product called cachectin

17 The tumour marker CEA
   A Is normally produced in the embryo from mesodermal tissues
   B Is elevated in up to 90% of patients with colorectal cancer
   C Is a useful screening tool for gastrointestinal cancer
   D The level of serum CEA is a poor marker of tumour mass
   E Correlates well with the Duke staging of colorectal cancer

18 The tumour marker AFP
   A Is an oncofetoprotein
   B Is a glycoprotein
   C Is elevated commonly in cases of seminoma of the testis
   D Is elevated commonly in cases of hepatocellular carcinoma
   E May, if measured serially, lead to a false sense of security when treating testicular malignancy

19 The following tumour markers and malignancies are correctly associated
   A CA-125: ovarian cancer
   B CEA: lung cancer
   C Neurone-specific enolase: lung cancer
   D AFP: seminoma of the testis
   E HCG: seminoma of the testis

20 The following are pre-neoplastic conditions
   A Xeroderma pigmentosa
   B Von Recklinghausen's disease
   C Ataxia telangiectasia
   D Retinoblastoma
   E X-linked agammaglobulinaemia

21 Tumour cell kinetics
   A Neoplastic cells divide more rapidly than normal cells
   B Neoplastic change results in a shortening of the cell cycle time
   C The majority of cells in a neoplasm are not in the replicative pool
   D Tumour growth is due to an imbalance between cell formation and cell death
   E Approximately 75% of neoplastic cells are lost from the replicative pool by death, shedding or differentiation

ONCOLOGY – Answers

1 **A** = True **B** = False **C** = True **D** = True **E** = False

Chemical carcinogens may produce neoplastic change by binding to, or chemically reacting with, the nucleotides of the DNA molecule. Initiation is the first step in neoplastic change, in which the DNA structure is irreversibly altered. It requires subsequent promotion of the cell in order to exert the changes caused by the alteration in the genome. Some chemicals, such as the aniline dyes, require conversion to become oncogenic and are not in themselves carcinogenic.

2 **A** = False **B** = False **C** = True **D** = True **E** = False

Promoter substances act by increasing cellular metabolism or cellular product formation, they do not alter the DNA structure of the cell. While it is true that initiation and promotion may occur many years apart, it must follow in the order of initiation first followed by promotion. Carcinogens are thought to act by causing misreading of the DNA sequences responsible for growth factor synthesis. Repair of damaged DNA structure is a highly efficient process, only when this fails does malignant change occur. This is exemplified by the conditions in which this process fail, such as xeroderma pigmentosa, when malignant tumours may be produced by the genetic changes induced by a diagnostic radiographic examination.

3 **A** = False **B** = True **C** = True **D** = False **E** = False

Polycyclic aromatic hydrocarbons require activation by the cellular microsomal enzymes to induce initiation of the cell. Ultimate carcinogens appear to be able to induce malignant change without the action of any other factor. They act as both initiator and promoter. Polycyclic aromatic hydrocarbons are strongly electrophilic chemicals. Polycyclic aromatic hydrocarbons are implicated in many cancers, particularly lung cancer, as they are found in cigarette smoke.

4 **A** = True **B** = False **C** = False **D** = True **E** = True

The formation of bladder tumours by aromatic amine compounds is a lengthy process. The compound is ingested and hydroxylated, producing a carcinogen, this is then detoxified by conjugation with glucuronic acid and excreted by the kidneys. In the bladder urinary glucuronidase reverses the conjugation releasing the carcinogen. In species lacking this urinary enzyme, such as rats, bladder tumours do not occur. These compounds are ultimate carcinogens, acting as its own initiator and promoter.

5 **A** = True **B** = True **C** = False **D** = True **E** = False

Part of the process of ultraviolet radiation-induced malignancy is related to reduction in cell mediated immunity, by unknown processes, related to the radiation. Xeroderma pigmentosa, Fanconi's anaemia, ataxia telangectasia and Bloom's syndrome are examples of conditions in which there is defective DNA repair, Wiskott–Aldrich syndrome is a condition of impaired immunity, thrombocytopaenia and eczema. Two theories of ultraviolet-induced malignancy are based on the formation of dimers and/or the interaction of free radicals of oxygen and water with the genome. Chronic myeloid leukaemia is almost never associated with radiation, unlike all the other leukaemias.

68 ONCOLOGY – Answers

6 A = False B = True C = False D = True E = False

The human papilloma virus is a DNA virus, not an RNA virus. Extracts of HPV genetic material have been found in over 90% of the squamous cell carcinomas of the cervix, of which 70% belong to the subclasses HPV-16 and HPV-18. Human papilloma virus has been implicated in neoplasia by its isolation in malignant cells as it has yet to be propagated in cell cultures.

7 A = True B = True C = False D = True E = False

Antibodies against the Epstein–Barr virus are found in every case of African Burkitt's lymphoma. Chronic parasitaemia, particularly with malaria, predisposes to the formation of African Burkitt's lymphoma. The virus causes proliferation within the B class of lymphocytes. There is a striking geographic distribution of neoplasms produced by this virus. The neoplastic change in the B cell is caused by a specific translocation: t(8;14).

8 A = True B = True C = True D = True E = True

V-oncs found in oncogenic viruses are thought to be normal cellular genes which have become incorporated into the viral genome during cellular reproduction. Hence, the cellular proto-oncogenes, c-onc, are genes which are responsible for the production of normal cellular constituents or growth factors. It is only when these proto-oncogenes become translocated to another location or are altered structurally that neoplastic change occurs.

9 A = True B = False C = True D = True E = True

Cellular proto-oncogenes are responsible for the formation of enzymes or cell structures such as receptors for cellular messengers. When they are translocated to a position adjacent to a promoter gene the production of the proto-oncogene product is increased dramatically leading to cell self-stimulation to grow and reproduce. The translocation for Burkitt's lymphoma is t(8;14) whereas chronic myeloid leukaemia has the Philadelphia chromosome t(9;22). Anti-oncogenes are believed to inhibit cell proliferation and hence inactivation of these genes cause, at least in theory, a loss of the normal inhibition of unchecked proliferation.

10 A = True B = False C = True D = False E = False

Retinoblastoma is an example of a neoplasm resulting from the loss of influence of anti-oncogenes. The gene in this case is referred to as the *Rb* locus. In order for the cells to proliferate both the DNA strands must lose the *Rb* locus. In the familial form there is an autosomally dominant loss of one of the two loci. In the sporadic form both loci must be deactivated for the cell to become neoplastic.

11 A = True B = True C = False D = False E = True

In neoplasms in which the DNA structure has been mapped, for example African Burkitt's lymphoma, all of the cells possess the same genome, including the translocation responsible for the neoplastic change. Initiation is synonymous with mutagenesis and involves an irreversible change in the genome. Autonomous cell activity is a feature of neoplasia but is due to aberrant enzyme or product formation and not strictly a feature of a 'genetic disease' *per se*.

ONCOLOGY – Answers

12 A = True   B = False   C = True   D = True   E = True

Benign tumours cause their effects by the fact of their location. They may produce hormones, cause pressure on adjacent structures, ulcerate and bleed if close to a body surface or cavity or outgrow their blood supply and necrose. These effects depend upon the size of the tumour and its site. Cachexia has been blamed upon chronic infection in the compromised host and/or the production of hormones such as cachectin by the immunocompetent cells. It is, however, not a factor of the energy required to sustain a growing malignancy. Malignant neoplasms produce effects upon the body unrelated to the tumour itself. These are called paraneoplastic syndromes.

13 A = True   B = False   C = True   D = True   E = False

Hypoglycaemia is due to the production of insulin-like polypeptides, and occurs in fibrosarcomas and other mesenchymal tumours. Hypercalcaemia occurs in many malignancies, including renal and bronchogenic carcinomas. This is thought to be due to the production of PTH-like peptides. Cushing's syndrome is produced by ACTH-like peptides and occurs with bronchogenic and pancreatic malignancies. Dermatomyositis occurs in conjuction with bronchogenic and breast cancers.

14 A = True   B = True   C = True   D = False   E = False

Only a small percentage of patients with malignant disease exhibit symptoms of a paraneoplastic syndrome. The tumour may produce hormones with activities similar to parathyroid hormone and ACTH. The reason for this aberrant hormone production appears to be derepression of normally quiescent portions of the genome; as clearly the genome must possess facilities for the synthesis of all of the cell constituents and peptides for all of the cells of the body. While it is true that serum calcium levels may increase in the presence of osseous involvement, it is also true that neoplasms have the ability to synthesize PTH-like peptides. The pathogenesis of myasthenia in malignant disease is not clear and hypotheses include antibody formation and/or toxic metabolites, although neither have been proved.

15 A = False   B = True   C = True   D = False   E = False

Hypercalcaemia is the commonest feature of the paraneoplastic syndromes. Its cause may be due to bone destruction by either primary osseous or secondary bone involvement. It may also be due to the production of parathyroid hormone-like peptides by malignant cells in non-osseous sites. TGF-α has an effect on osteoclasts causing increased bone destruction. Hypercalcaemia secondary to malignant disease is very difficult to treat and is often refractory to the therapies employed in Cushing's disease.

16 A = True   B = True   C = False   D = False   E = True

The cachexia of malignant disease is a subject of controversy. While it seems to be related to the tumour burden of the host, it is certainly not due to increased nutritional demands incurred by the growing tumour. It may be related to chronic low-grade infection in the host caused by immunosuppression, and also to a central reduction in appetite, by processes unknown. Cachectin, a macrophage product known also as TNF-α, has been implicated in the wasting associated with malignant disease.

ONCOLOGY – Answers

17 **A** = False **B** = True **C** = False **D** = False **E** = True

Carcinoembryonic antigen is produced in the fetus from ectodermal structures. In series the rate of elevated CEA in patients with colorectal cancer has been found to be 60–90%. While it is elevated in patients with cancers of the gastrointestinal tract and breast it is also found to be raised in several other conditions and even in healthy smokers. In the presence of a gastrointestinal malignancy the level of serum CEA is related to the tumour mass and even correlates with the stage of the tumour within the Duke classification.

18 **A** = True **B** = True **C** = False **D** = False **E** = False

Alpha foetoprotein is both a glycoprotein and an oncofetoprotein. It is produced by normal tissues during the foetal period. In the adult elevated serum levels are found in non-seminiferous testicular and hepatic malignancies. Levels also rise in liver damage from cirrhosis and hepatitis. Its level rises in germ cell tumours and affords an excellent marker for response to cancer therapy and the detection of recurrence.

19 **A** = True **B** = True **C** = True **D** = False **E** = False

CA-125 is a specific tumour marker for ovarian malignancy. CEA levels rise in gastrointestinal, lung, and breast malignancy. Neurone-specific enolase levels rise in cancers of the lung and neuroblastoma. Alpha fetoprotein levels rise in non-seminiferous malignancy of the testis and hepatocellular tumours. Human chorionic gonadotrophic hormone levels rise is non-seminiferous malignancy of the testis and trophoblastic tumours.

20 **A** = True **B** = True **C** = True **D** = False **E** = True

All of the examples in this question have an increased malignant potential. Von Recklinghausen's disease is an example of the phakomatoses. Xeroderma pigmentosa and ataxia telangiectasia are examples of conditions in which DNA repair mechanisms are defective and hence the DNA structure is unstable. In X-linked agammaglobulinaemia there is immune deficiency leading to increased cases of leukaemias and lymphomas. Retinoblastoma is an example of the heritable malignancies.

21 **A** = False **B** = False **C** = True **D** = True **E** = True

It is neither true that neoplastic cells replicate themselves more rapidly or have a greater proportion of their number in the replicative pool at any time. In fact the converse is true. The reason for the excessive growth encountered in neoplasms is that the growth is disordered and cell proliferation exceeds that of cell loss. In normal tissues cells reproduce to replace lost members, in the neoplasm the cells keep reproducing whether other cells in the tumour are lost or not.